HISTORY OF OPHTHALMOLOGY 6

ACADEMIA OPHTHALMOLOGICA INTERNATIONALIS

History of Ophthalmology 6

Sub auspiciis
Academiae Ophthalmologicae Internationalis

Editor HAROLD E. HENKES
Geervliet, The Netherlands

Associate Editor CLAUDIA ZRENNER
Tübingen, Germany

Associate Editor DANIEL M. ALBERT
Madison, Wisconsin, USA

Kluwer Academic Publishers
Dordrecht / Boston / London

ISBN 0-7923-3101-X

Published by Kluwer Academic Publishers,
P.O. Box 17, 3300 AA Dordrecht, The Netherlands.

Kluwer Academic Publishers incorporates the publishing programmes of
D. Reidel, Martinus Nijhoff, Dr W. Junk and MTP Press.

Sold and distributed in the U.S.A. and Canada
by Kluwer Academic Publishers,
101 Philip Drive, Norwell, MA 02061, U.S.A.

In all other countries, sold and distributed
by Kluwer Academic Publishers Group,
P.O. Box 322, 3300 AH Dordrecht, The Netherlands.

History of Ophthalmology, Volume 6
Reprinted from *Documenta Ophthalmologica*, Vol. 86, No. 2 (1994).

Already published:
History of Ophthalmology, Volume 1
1988 – ISBN 0-89838-366-8
History of Ophthalmology, Volume 2
1989 – ISBN 0-7923-0273-7
History of Ophthalmology, Volume 3
1990 – ISBN 0-7923-0826-3
History of Ophthalmology, Volume 4
1991 – ISBN 0-7923-1545-6
History of Ophthalmology, Volume 5
1993 – ISBN 0-7923-2053-0

Printed in the Netherlands (on acid-free paper)

Documenta Ophthalmologica **86**: 111–122, 1994.

Prominent ophthalmologists who suffered from acute glaucoma

FREDERICK C. BLODI
Iowa City, Iowa

Key words: History of ophthalmology, Glaucoma, Pagenstecher, Wagner, Laqueur, Javal

Abstract. We know of at least four ophthalmologists who suffered from glaucoma had to be treated. I would like to discuss them according to degree of severity of the disease. The first ophthalmologist was hardly bothered at all whereas the fourth one became blind in both eyes.

Alexander Pagenstecher (1828–1879)

Alexander Pagenstecher was a member of an old and venerable patrician family in Hessen-Nassau (Fig. 1). He was the son of a senior forest official and was born in a little village near Wiesbaden. He studied medicine as of 1846 at the universities of Giessen, Heidelberg and Würzberg. He graduated in Würzburg in 1849 and went to Paris in 1851 where he studied ophthalmology under Desmarres and Sichel.

In 1852 he was appointed assistant at the Civilian Hospital of Wiesbaden. He soon acquired a large general and ophthalmologic practice. In 1853 he married the daughter of the Würzburg professor of botany, Heller.

He made repeated trips to Berlin to visit A. von Graefe, also to London to see Bowman and Critchett. He had excellent relationships to W. Hess in Mainz and Horner in Zurich. He soon decided to practice ophthalmology only.

Pagenstecher was a skillful surgeon and a successful physician, especially treating external eye diseases with the specific yellow mercury oxide ointment, which for a long time was referred to as the Pagenstecher ointment.

In 1853 a small eye clinic was founded in Wiesbaden. The building was enlarged in 1857 and moved into a bigger house in 1860 (Fig. 2). A new clinic was erected in 1905.[1]

Pagenstecher published clinical observations which summarized the experience gathered in his clinic. His papers were mainly concerned with sympathetic ophthalmia, the indications for enucleation, iridodesis, glaucoma and intracapsular cataract extraction. He personally performed more than 2000 cataract operations. He had a distinguished career and was appointed Hofrat (Fig. 3).

He developed pleuritis and hemoptysis which forced him to reduce his practice. In 1878 he had an acute glaucomatous attack in the right eye and

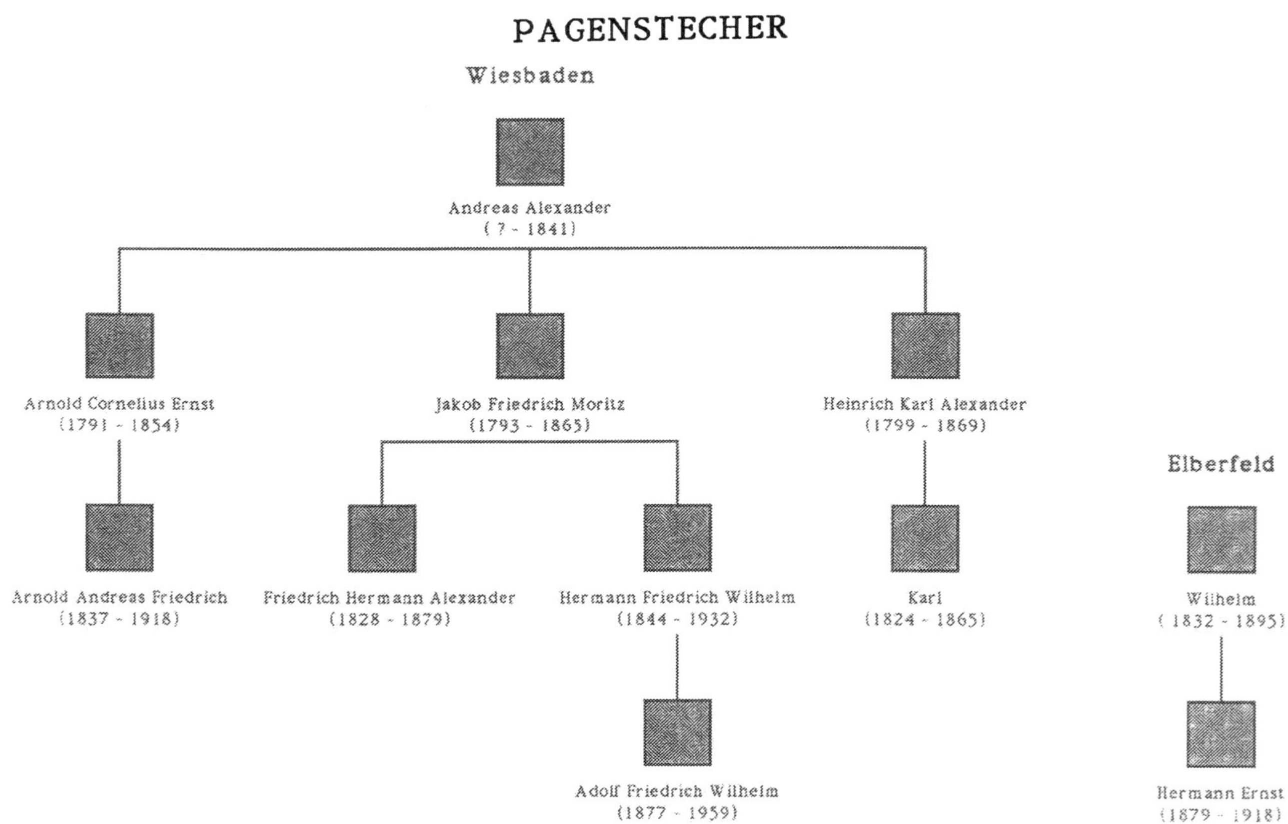

Fig. 1 Family tree of the Wiesbaden and the Elberfeld branches of the Pagenstecher family. Many of the members were ophthalmologists.

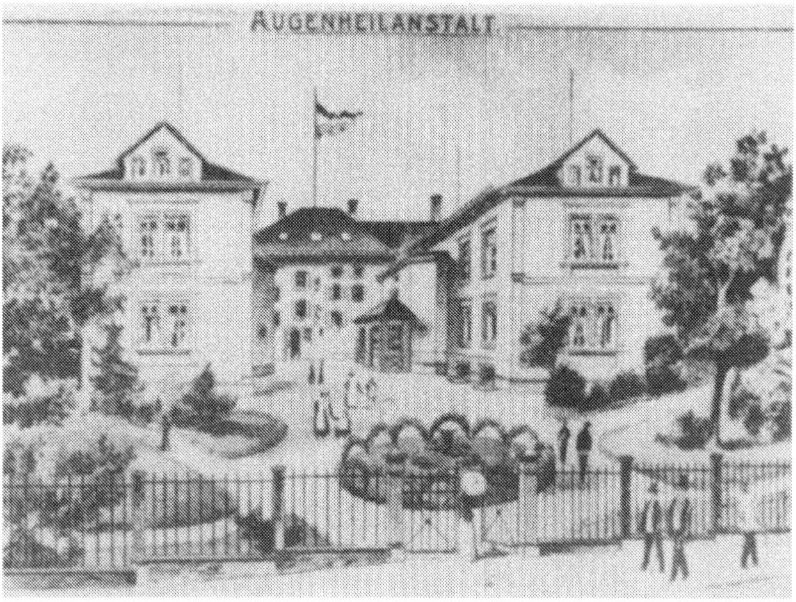

Fig. 2. The eye clinic of Wiesbaden.

was immediately operated on by his brother, Hermann, who performed a complete iridectomy. No visual deficit remained.

Pagenstecher died shortly thereafter from an unusual hunting accident. When mounting a coach his gun accidentally went off and perforated his skull. He expired two days later on New Year's Eve of 1879.[2]

His brother, Hermann, later Geheimrat (Fig. 4), then became the director of the eye institute. He was followed by Hermann's son, Adolf.

Wilhelm Wagner (1836–1915)

Wagner[3] was born in Prussia and trained in Berlin. However, most of his professional life was spent in Odessa, the Ukrainian city on the Black Sea. He became there the chief of the Municipal Eye Hospital in 1888.

A university had been founded in Odessa in 1864 and a medical school was established 1897. The Municipal Eye Hospital had been erected in 1875 and its first director was Heinrich Stieder, a German ophthalmologist who had settled in Russia. Stieder died in 1889 and Wagner became his successor. The hospital was enlarged and encompassed then 80 beds.

Wagner was a senior staff physician in the Prussian Army during the war of 1870–71. He was awarded the Knighthood of the Iron Cross. When he retired, he returned to Berlin to take up private practice, but he soon

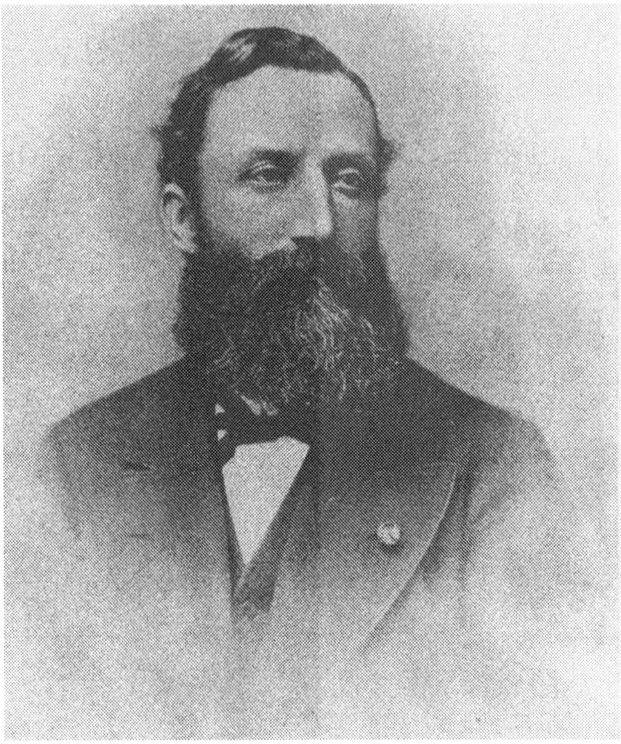

Fig. 3. Hofrat Alexander Pagenstecher.

became too sick to keep on working. His successor at the Odessa Hospital was Dr. Walter.

Wagner experienced his first glaucomatous attack in the left eye in 1877 when he was 44 years old. He had a history of migraine in his youth (so did his mother) and these attacks had started at the age of 17. They occurred mainly when he got cold and would affect either one or the other half of his head. He frequently had to use morphine to interrupt the attack, but he never had nausea and usually the attack improved after a short sleep.

Otherwise, he had been healthy and had good vision. The right eye was emmetropic and the left eye had a myopic astigmatism and floaters which he thought could be due to a fencing injury when he was a student. He had good accommodation and showed pronounced senile arcus in both corneas.

Already in the summer of 1875 he had noticed that the left pupil was somewhat wider and reacted poorly to light. Vision and accommodation remained normal though the eye felt somewhat hard.

The attack in 1877 occurred in December and was associated with foggy vision, colored rings around lights, a dilated and rigid pupil, deep pain

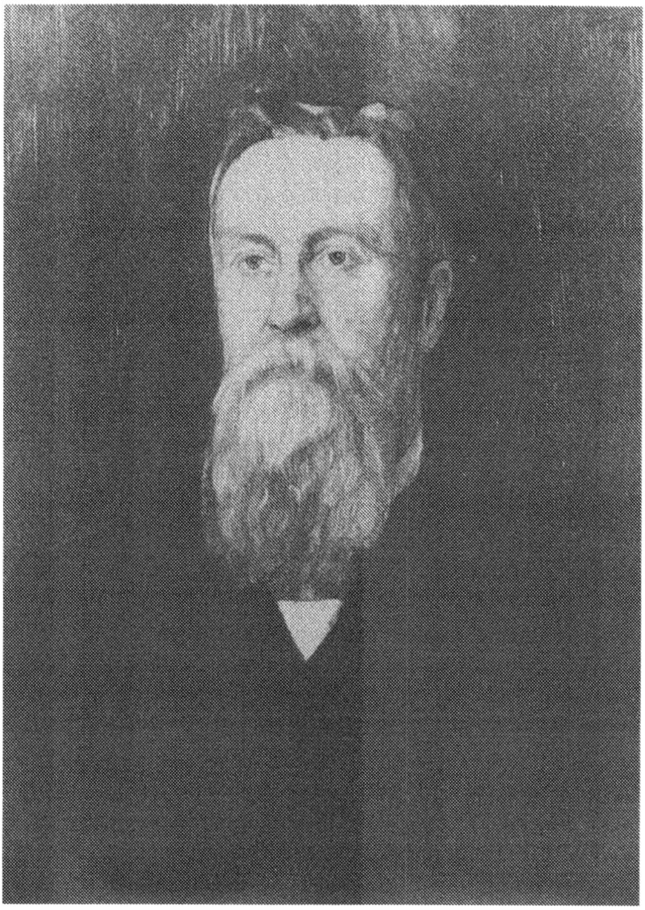

Fig. 4. Geheimrat Hermann Pagenstecher.

around the eye and a hardening of the eyeball. The attack occurred in the evening during a conference and was relieved after a good night's sleep.

The attacks became more and more frequent and occurred mainly after reading or writing, sometimes during an operation. The administration of eserine relieved the attacks promptly.

In 1878, an iridectomy was performed on the left eye by his colleague, Dr. Schmid. After that he had no more glaucomatous attacks, but suffered from slight photophobia and somewhat reduced dark adaptation in the left eyc.

Wagner had always been interested in glaucoma and was convinced that iridectomy could cure every patient with this disease. He first maintained this point of view in a short note which was published in 1891.[4]

At the 25th International Congress of Medicine in Moscow (1897), he reported before Section XI (Ophthalmology) on August 11 his statistics and surgical treatment of glaucoma.[5] This was the fifth session of this section and represented presentation #27. The session was presided by J. Hirschberg. Here Wagner reported that among 74,930 eye patients (seen within nine years in Odessa) there were 1227 with glaucoma (1.63%) and among them were 476 men and 751 women; in a previous report he found a prevalence of 2.09% glaucoma patients and a relative higher frequency among Jews.

In 1883,[6] he reported on some aspects of glaucoma followed by a report on his own attack. In this paper he also reported on seeing 20,000 eye patients of which nearly half were Jews, though they only represented 27% of the entire population. Among 410 patients with glaucoma, 62 of them were Jews.

He returned to this theme in 1901 in a larger publication[7] and again claimed that iridectomy is the best operation against all types of glaucoma.

Wagner never had any attacks in his right eye and the left eye remained cured all his life, i.e. for nearly forty years.

Ludwig Laqueur (1837–1909)

Laqueur[8] (whole original name was apparently Herz[9]) was born in Silesia which was then a Prussian province. He attended medical school in Berlin graduating in 1860. In 1861 he became Graefe's assistant at the eye clinic. After he finished his training he went in 1863 to Paris to work with Liebreich. In 1869 he obtained the French medical degree and licence. He moved to Lyon and opened a practice for eye diseases. During the Franco-Prussian War of 1870–71, he joined the Prussian Army and was appointed chief physician of a Prussian division and worked in a military hospital. After the war he returned to Lyon, but in 1872 was called to Strasbourg and appointed professor and chairman of the eye department at that university (Fig. 5).

Laqueur made a number of valuable contributions to ophthalmic practice. His most important paper was probably the one on physostigmine which he introduced for the first time as a medical treatment for glaucoma in 1877.[10]

Since the age of 30 he suffered from the prodromal signs of a glaucomatous attack. In his paper on the prodromal stages of glaucoma,[11] he gives an excellent survey of the first symptoms of an angle closure attack. This paper is not only based on his experience with a great number of patients, but also on his own personal history, though he does not say so explicitly in this article.

Laqueur was extremely reluctant to let anybody know about his eye condition. He wrote about his own history in September/October 1902, but requested that it not be published until he died. Indeed, the paper appeared posthumously in 1909.[12]

Laqueur first states that he is of Jewish descent and he believes that this

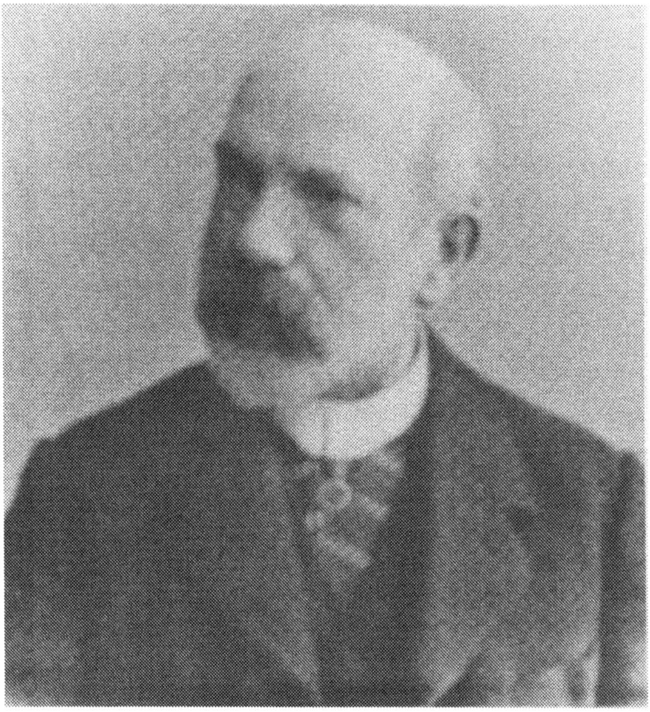

Fig. 5. Ludwig Laqueur.

race has a strong disposition to develop angle closure glaucoma. His paternal grandmother had been blind for thirty years because of acute glaucoma, but no other family member had a positive history. He had been red-green blind since birth, but was otherwise emmetropic and had good vision. He did complain about photophobia and suffered from chronic recurrent conjunctivitis for which he used a 1.5% silver nitrate solution. He wore sunglasses whenever illumination was too bright. He developed an induced astigmatism at the age of 33 probably due to the pressure by a pince-nez (0.75 D × 180° O.D.)

Laqueur had the first prodromal attack in 1847. It had been a long and weary day in the operating room. One patient on whom he performed a blepharoplasty had severe bleeding and recovered only slowly. When he went home, he noticed foggy vision in the right eye and during his late lunch he had the same symptom in his left eye. He also noticed rainbow colors around light and palpating his eyes he thought that they had become hard. He recovered the same day.

He had two to three recurrences in the left eye, the last one in March 1880 after the right eye had been operated on. He had many hundred attacks in the right eye. These occurred mainly after psychological upsets, stress and other unpleasant events.

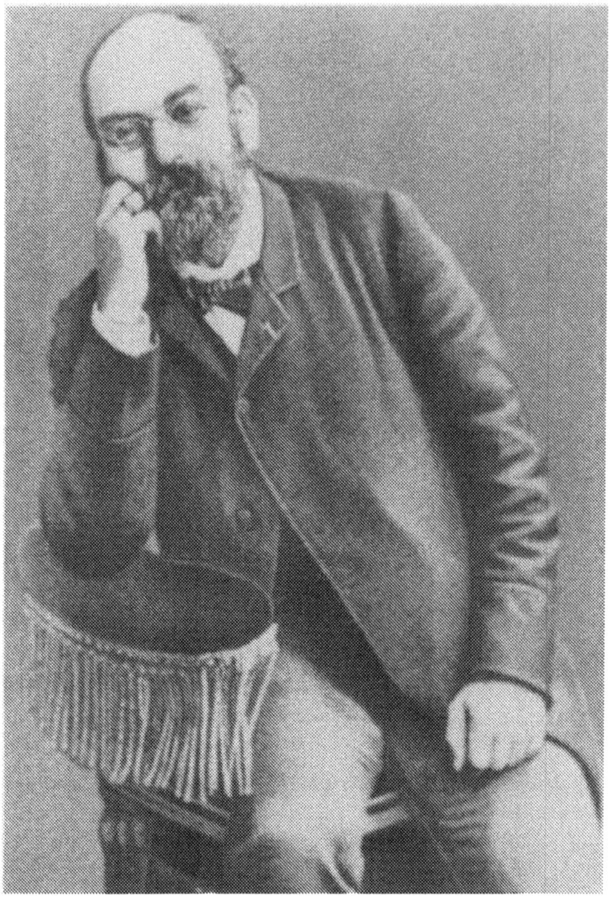

Fig. 6. Louis-Emile Javal (print by Sauvanaud).

During the winter 1874/75, the attacks were still separated by relatively long intervals (two to three weeks). However, they became more frequent and often he had three attacks daily in the right eye, some of them lasting an hour or more. He even had attacks during the night when he suddenly would wake up. The rainbow colors became less vivid and he never had any actual pain, nor were the eyes injected.

During an attack the vision in the affected eye would drop to 3/4 or 1/10. He did not notice any field restrictions, but did realize that the attacks were triggered by anger, embarrassment, rage, hearing sentimental music or watching a beautiful scene in the theater; they could also be elicited by hunger, bad ventilation of a room, etc.

As of 1876, he used physostigmine and it always worked. One drop was enough to cut the attack, but they, nevertheless, recurred.

Occasionally, the attack in the right eye would occur during an operation or a lecture and this nearly incapacitated him. In 1878, he visited for the first time Professor Horner in Zurich.

Horner told him to keep on using physostigmine, put him on a diet and advised him to take small doses of quinine.

During the summer of 1879, the condition was not worse, though he had now the disease for five years.

In November of that year he returned to Zurich and Horner found a change in the optic nerve. He called it 'not as diaphanous' as before, but he did not see any glaucomatous excavation. Visual acuity and field were normal.

On March 18, 1880 he was admitted to Horner's private clinic. He did not reveal his identity and his name remained unknown except to Horner and the head nurse. An iridectomy was performed on the right side using a keratome. As no local anesthetic was available at that time, the patient felt a slight burning sensation, but no real pain. He was put on bed rest for three days and then developed an attack in the left eye. Therefore, an iridectomy was also performed on the left side on March 25. This time he had severe postoperative pain and feared that a malignant glaucoma could develop. Morphine was injected and the situation improved.

Laqueur was discharged on April 4 and remained nine days in Zurich. He then went for 6 days to Baden Baden for a cure and returned 18 days later to Strasbourg and resumed full work. Vision in both eyes was good, about 3/4ths to 5/6ths with correction (a 3/4 diopter cylinder against the rule). He experienced only one slight further attack on the right side, but remained photophobic to sunlight.

The left coloboma was slightly visible because it was wider and somewhat displaced temporally. Laqueur became extremely self-conscious about this condition and acquired the habit to half-close his eyes. He also did not look into his colleagues' eyes when talking with them and developed folds on his forehead because he constantly tried to close partially his lids. He did not go to the Heidelberg congresses because he was afraid that people would notice his eye condition and ask him about his glaucoma. Nevertheless, the condition remained cured for more than twenty years.

Laqueur died in St. Margharita, near Nervi (close to Genoa).

Louis-Emile Javal (1839–1907)

Javal was born in Paris, the son of an influential and wealthy banker and industrialist.[13] He became first engineer and worked for onc ycar in a coal mine.

He became interested in strabismus because his father had a marked secondary exotropia (he had an esotropia operated on by Desmarres in 1846) and his sister was esotropic. He was fascinated by medicine and enrolled in the University of Paris. He graduated in 1868 dealing with strabismus.

Javal visited Graefe in Berlin and then served in the Franco-Prussian War. He became concerned with public health and was elected to the National Assembly.

He became director of a new ophthalmologic laboratory of the Sorbonne and published, among others, a manual on strabismus (1896).[14] Of greatest importance became his keratometer which made the ophthalmometer of Helmholtz a most useful and important clinical instrument.[15]

In 1881 he noted the first prodromal signs of an acute glaucoma in his right eye, but he was operated on only four years later and in 1886 the eye became blind. The first prodromal signs in the left eye appeared 1885 and he was not operated on until 1900 and this eye became blind the same year, though he had been transiently blind already in 1897 when he attended the court-martial in Rennes against Captain Dreyfus whom he passionately supported.

The first public discussion on his condition took place in 1901 when De Wecker gave a report to the annual meeting of the French Ophthalmological Society on the value of iridectomy in the treatment of glaucoma.[16] De Wecker polled the audience and also referred to 'an unfortunate colleague' who had become blind because the iridectomy had been performed too late.

Javal discussed the report and revealed that he was the 'unfortunate colleague'.[17] Javal had just turned 62 and mentioned that had he died at the age of 60 his case would have been a classical example of the effectiveness of miotics. He stated that the operation is quite useful performed early in the disease, but may have deplorable results when done later, especially after prolonged use of miotics. Miotics are a double-edged sword. Javal regretted not to have been put on atropine after the operation, as practiced by Graefe and recommended for him by Priestley-Smith.

De Wecker[18] concluded the discussion and first explained that not he, but his associate had operated on the right eye in 1885. Again, in 1900, De Wecker had to leave for Cairo and turned Javal over to Masselon, who advised against an operation. Javal turned to Priestley-Smith who performed an iridectomy and a sclerotomy on the left eye. The operations were executed well, but the progress of the disease could not be arrested. The operations were performed too late.

In the same session, Javal gives more details and enumerates the alleged mistakes perpetrated in the treatment of his glaucoma,[19] e.g., the iridectomy was done at 12:00 o'clock (not temporally as advised by Graefe), the operation were done too early (when there were only minimal signs and symptoms), the daily use of miotics masked a progress of the disease.

Javal then published a complete report on his disease.[20] From it we see that the eyes were frequently smothered with drops and many operations followed each other in quick succession. (Between February 7, 1900 and March 28 seven different operations were performed on the left eye). The right eye was enucleated on March 16, 1900. The histologic examination revealed a complete retinal detachment, retinal and subretinal hemorrhages. The iris was plastered against the cornea.

The left superior sympathetic ganglion was excised on June 25, 1900. De Wecker advised it on the basis of some reports from Romania. It did not change the condition of the eye.

Javal had consulted J. Jacobson when the latter visited Paris in 1886. Jacobson made some critical remarks about the rapidity with which one operation followed another.[21] On the other hand, Jacobson[22] and Hirschberg[23] criticized Javal that he did not choose one ophthalmologist on whom he could rely, that he did not return for follow-up examination, that he wanted to control his own treatment, that he delayed necessary operation, etc.

The blind Javal invented an armrest with a cogwheel device advancing the writing paper by 1 cm at the end of each line. This 'planchette scotographique' could be used by blind persons to write ordinary script.

Javal also published a monograph[24] in which he advised patients who were blind late in life, their families and their physicians. They should become as independent as possible and should remain gainfully employed. The book was translated into German, English and Esperanto. (Javal was a good friend of Zamenhof, the Polish ophthalmologist who invented and championed Esperanto.).

Javal died after a short illness from an abdominal tumor.

Notes

1. 100 Jahre Augenheilanstalt Wiesbaden; Wiesbaden 1956.
2. Obituaries: Anon: Klin. Monatsbl. f. Augenhk. 18:68, 1880. Horstmann: Centralbl. f. Augenhk. 4:25, 1880.
3. Obituary: Anon: Centralbl. f. Augenhk. 39:93, 1915.
4. Wagner, W.: St. Petersburg med. Wochenschr. May/June 1891 (Centralbl. f. Augenhk. 15:462, 1891).
5. Wagner, W.: Centralbl. f. Augenhk. 22:435, 1898.
6. Wagner, W.: Einiges über Glaucom im Anschluss an einen Bericht über meine Erkrankung an Glaucom; Arch. f. Ophth. 29, 2, 280, 1883.
7. Wagner, W.: Die Iridectomie hat zur Zeit als beste Operation gegen Glaucom aller klinischen Glaucom-Gruppen zu gelten, Klin. Monatsbl. f. Augenhk. 39, II, 558, 1901.
8. a) Obituaries: Hirschberg, J.; Centralbl. f. Augenhk. 33:157, 1909. Landolt, H.; Klin. Monatsbl. f. Augenhk. 47:536, 1909. Anon.; Arch. f. Augenhk. 63:134, 1909.
   b) Snyder, Ch.: Ludwig Laqueur, in: Our Ophthalmic Heritage; Little, Brown and Co., Boston, 1967, p. 131.
9. Bronner, A. (Strasbourg): Communication to the Hirschberg Society and the Francophone Society for Ophthalmologic History, Munich, January 19/20, 1990
10. Laqueur, L.: Ueber Atropin und Physostigmin und ihre Wirkung auf den intraocularen Druck; Arch. f. Ophth. 23, 3, 149, 1877.
11. Laqueur, L.: Geschichte meiner Glaukomerkrankung, Klin. Monatsbl. f. Augenhk. 47, 1, 639, 1909 (Translated by E. Jackson in Am. J. Ophth. 12:984, 1929).

13. Obituaries: J. Hirschberg: Centralbl. f. Augenhk, 31:61, 1907. Sulzer: Ann. d'ocul. 137:178, 1907. Tscherning: Klin. Monatsbl. f. Augenhk. 45:375, 1907. Terrien, F.: Arch. d'opht. 27:65, 1907. Anon: Recueil d'opht. 1907, p. 63.
14. Javal, E.: Manuel théorique et pratique du strabisme; Paris 1896.
15. Javal, E.: Mémoires d'ophtalmométrie; Paris 1890.
16. De Wecker, L.: Valeur de l'iridectomie dans le glaucome, Ann. d'ocul. 125:421, 1901.
17. Javal, E.: Ann. d'ocul. 125:445, 1901.
18. De Wecker, L.: Ann. d'ocul. 125:456, 1901.
19. Javal, E.: Ann. d'ocul. 126:143, 1901.
20. Javal, E.: Auto-observations de glaucome (cas malheureux); Ann. d'ocul. 126:161, 1901.
21. Jacobson, J.: Briefe an Fachgenossen (Margarethe Quidde, editor), Königsberg 1899, p. 109.
22. Jacobson, J.: ibidem, p. 125.
23. Hirchberg. J.: Die Augenheilkunde in der Neuzeit (chapter XXIII); Julius Springer, Berlin 1916, p. 540.
24. Javal, E.: Entre aveugles; Masson et Cie, Paris 1903.

Address for correspondence: Frederick C. Blodi, MD, Department of Ophthalmology, University of Iowa, Iowa City, IA 522 42, USA

Documenta Ophthalmologica **86**: 123–151, 1994.

Vision and cognition in the natural philosophy of Albert the Great (Albertus Magnus)

PETER THEISS & OTTO-JOACHIM GRÜSSER
Department of Physiology, Freie University, Berlin, Germany

Dedicated to Sir John Eccles on the occasion of his 90th birthday in deep respect and grateful appreciation of his support of post-war German neuroscience three and four decades ago.

Key words: History of Ophthalmology, Cognition, Vision, Albertus Magnus

Abstract. Albert the Great (*Albertus Magnus*, ca. 1197–1280) descended from a nobleman's family in Upper Suebia and studied natural philosophy and theology at the University of Padova, where he joined the Dominican order. Confronted with Aristotelian thought mainly in its Arabic modification (Avicenna, Al-Farabi, Averroes, Alhazen, Costa ben Luca and others) from his days in Padova, he elaborated in several books on the principles of natural philosophy, biology, brain and sense functions and psychology in addition to his theological and exegetic works. His observations and concepts on vision are discussed in detail. It is pointed out that Albert discovered some phenomena of vision not before known such as vestibular nystagmus and rod monochromacy, i.e. total colour blindness accompanied by photophobia. Based on clinical observations Albert also postulated a decussation of the optic nerve fibres at the optic chiasm. Albert's concept of higher order cognitive function is discussed and some of his explanations of dreams and neuropsychiatric disease on the basis of his cognitive model are mentioned. Albert's thoughts on vision and other sense perceptions, higher brain functions and cognition are considered as progressive elaborations of Galenic concepts as adapted by some Patristic theologians and the Arabic natural scientists and philosophers of the 9th–11th century.

Introduction

The thirteenth century marked a turning point in the history of Western thought. Becoming more acquainted and familiar with the body of Aristotelian writings and his Arabian commentators, the Latin world underwent a period of profound transformation in the theological and philosophical foundation of its way of thinking and self-perception. Assimilating the Aristotelian approach to problem-solving resulted not only in the increasing autonomy of natural philosophy, but also gave way to a thorough investigation of sense perception as the basis of human knowledge. Theories of vision, the sense modality providing the main source of empirical data, received a high degree of interest.

Albert the Great (about 1197–1280, 'Albert of Lauingen', *Albertus Magnus*), a Dominican friar, played a leading role in this process; he can be considered as one of the most important scholars of the century. Together with his pupil *Thomas Aquinas* (1225–1274), he is referred to today as the *Founder of Christian Aristotelianism.*[1] This statement tends to obscure the obstacles Albert had to overcome in bringing his contemporaries to accept the Aristotelian approach to the natural sciences. The ruling doctrine of the time was Augustinian and Neoplatonic, rooted in a long Patristic and Scholastic tradition which hindered a smooth transition of scholarly thinking to an empirical scientific approach. Since 12th-century Christian theology and anthropology was dominated by doctrines combining Neoplatonic and mystic thought, it was a great struggle for Aristotelian Latin writers to smooth out the contradictions and make different ideological principles compatible which to some extent just did not go together. In 13th-century Paris, the centre of the western Medieval intellectual community, Aristotles' books appeared on the Index several times. Conservative theologians were particularly concerned about the Aristotelian interpretation of *Averroes* (1126–1198). This Arab philosopher and physician from Cordoba (Andalusia) had elaborated upon a consequent explanation of Aristotle's philosophy, thereby denying that the individual human soul was immortal. Such ideas were a threat to clerical power and could not be allowed to stand without a forceful rebuttal. Despite his preference for Aristotelian philosophy, Albertus Magnus allied himself, at least in part, to the theological forces against Averroes, while in his natural philosophy he did not wish to disagree with the main concepts of this and other Arabic Aristotelians.[2]

In England, the situation was slightly different. By the middle of the 12th century, Platonist philosophers had begun to emphasize the mathematical aspects of Plato's thinking in natural philosophy as well as its applicability to practical and technological problems.[3] When the translations of Aristotle's writings appeared, they could be discussed relatively freely in Oxford, and censorship was restricted to the period of *suspendium clericorum* (1209–1214) during which the teachers of Oxford were forced into exile, many of them moving to Paris.[4] Also in the following generations this city remained a place of interest for scholars from the British isles and an intellectual centre participating in the struggle with Aristotle's thoughts as interpreted by Arabic and Jewish philosophers. During his first period of study and teaching in the decade following 1240, *Roger Bacon* (about 1214–1292) also came to Paris and met Albert the Great on this occasion. On his return to Oxford, Bacon could look back upon a venerable tradition of teachers in his home country, like *Robert Grosseteste* (about 1168–1253) and *Adam Marsh* (ca. 1195–1259), who tried to apply empirical aspects to natural philosophy. The years in Paris were the beginning of a long and overall productive competition between Roger Bacon, who later joined the Franciscan order, and Albertus Magnus, the intellectual forerunner of the Dominicans. While Albert became an unquestioned authority in his order, Roger Bacon had to overcome serious criticism on the part of his superiors. In 1257 *Saint*

Bonaventura (1221–1274), the General of the Franciscans, forbade Roger Bacon to write, and after 1278 indexed his books with the result that Bacon was imprisoned for 14 years.[5] Thus in the intellectual dispute between the *doctor universalis* Albert and the *doctor mirabilis* Roger Bacon the working conditions were rather different for the two protagonists of 13th century sciences. With respect to natural philosophy both favoured an empirical approach, a *scientia experimentalis*, which included sensory experience and internal 'illumination' as sources for natural sciences. They relied on careful observations in biology or optics but also accepted astrology and to a moderate extent even magic as sources for natural philosophy. Accordingly one must take care not to project the modern scientific approach to nature onto the 13th century 'empiricists'.[6]

Albert's biography

Although there can be no doubt that Albert was older than Bacon, we can still not give a precise birth date. It is most likely that he was born around the year 1197 as the son of a lesser nobleman, Marquard of Lauingen, in the town of Lauingen on the Danube river close to Ulm in Upper Suebia. As the offspring of a knightly family which had been in the service of *Frederic Babarossa*, Albert was in all likelihood expected to pursue a military career.[7]

We know little about his youth, but it is probable that he attended the Latin school in Augsburg. In his books on natural philosophy he repeatedly mentioned observations he had made as a boy along the Danube.[8] In 1222 Albert went to Padova and studied the liberal arts at the incipient university for the following 6 or 7 years. Since medicine was closely associated with the liberal arts in *Padova*, Albert must have acquired at least the basis of contemporary medical knowledge.[9] Here he presumably encountered texts of Aristotelian and Arabic philosophy for the first time. It was also in Italy around 1223 that he joined the Dominican order, founded in 1216 by *Saint Dominicus* and confirmed by Pope *Honorius III* in 1216 when *Jordan of Saxonia* was the General of the order. Today one wonders how someone interested in natural philosophy could join an order so restricting personal freedom. To understand this decision one should realize what progressive intentions the mendicant orders had had since their founding in the early decades of the 13th century.[10] The church had some difficulties in integrating the new intellectually active orders since they not only expressed a certain social protest, but also took on an important part of the educational system and dared to take new approaches to philosophical inquiries.

Albert spent the next two decades in the province of Teutonia (Germany), lecturing, travelling and observing very carefully the details of nature on his journeys. In 1228 Albert became lector of the Dominicans in Cologne and in 1243 the Dominicans sent him to Paris, where he first lectured at the university and graduated to *doctor theologiae*. In 1245 he took over the chair of the Dominicans as magister (*Regent Master*) of theology. Throughout this period Albert was particularly interested in the 'new learning' and read Arabic and Jewish (e.g. Moses Maimonides) scripts that interpreted Aristotle. He also took part in antisemitic actions, however, as in the condemnation of the Talmud. It seems to have been in Paris that Albert discovered his life's ideal: to make the entire corpus of Aristotelian scripts accessible to his contemporaries, to comment on them as *Avicenna* (980–1037) had done two centuries before, to fill in the gaps left by Aristotle and correct him where he had been mistaken. The *Summa de creaturis*, the first work in which Albert dealt with sense physiology and perception, originated from the time in Paris. It still shows the strong influence of Augustian thinking.[11] Albert met not only *Roger Bacon* in Paris, but most likely also *Thomas Aquinas*, who became his pupil. Returning with Thomas to Cologne in 1248, Albert established the *studium generale* of his Dominican order there. His school for friars soon became a place of high intellectual repute, existing for many generations into the time *Heymericus de Campo* (1395–1460) and *Nicolaus Cusanus* (1401–1464) studied Albert's writings.[12] In Cologne Albert continued his systematic exposition of Peripatetic natural philosophy. Various facts indicate the mutual affinity that was to develop between Albert and the citizens of Cologne. More than once he was asked to settle a dispute between the townspeople and clerical authorities. The high esteem in which he was held is also reflected in the myth that it was Albert who worked out the plans for constructing the cathedral of Cologne (begun in 1248).

In 1254 when he was elected *Prior provincialis* of the Dominicans in *Teutonia* (Germany) Albertus Magnus became somewhat distracted from his studies. Nevertheless he still found the time to continue his philosophical work and to accomplish his major contribution to psychology (*De anima*).[13] As *Prior provincialis* he was called to the court of Pope *Alexander IV*, residing then at Anagni, where he had to defend his order in the struggle against strong anti-mendicant attacks from within the more traditional powers of the church. In the year 1260 Albert was forced to take on a duty he never grew very fond of, namely as bishop to reorganize the run-down episcopate of Regensburg. Two years later he sought release, but once again was hindered in dedicating himself totally to his scientific work, as he received the order to propagate a new crusade by preaching in the German-speaking countries. In the fall of 1263 he withdrew to the Dominican monastery of Würzburg, where he continued his studies, as was also the case after he moved to the Dominican monastery of Strasbourg in 1267.

When Albert returned to Cologne in 1270 he was still highly involved in a number of clerical duties and in church politics. Till 1280, the last year of his life, he remained an intellectually active philosopher and theologian, who had acquired a remarkable reputation in Western Europe. Despite the fact that Albert was held in the highest repute and admiration by his contemporaries, his reputation later became somewhat obscured by that of his pupil

Thomas Aquinas, whom he had to defend in 1277 during the anti-Aristotelian attacks in Paris. *Dante Alighieri* (1265–1302) mentioned both of them in his *Divina Commedia* where Thomas speaks of Albert as his *brother and master.*[14] Thomas Aquinas' theology and moderate Aristotelism were easier to integrate into church orthodoxy than Albert's philosophy which contained at least a kernel of theological agnosticism.[15] It took more than 600 years until the canonization of Albert in 1931. Ten years later, in a period when the harmful effects of modern technology became more than evident, Albert was declared patron of the natural sciences by the Roman Catholic church.

Albert's *Opera omnia* were first published in Lyon by P. Jammy in 1651 and reprinted between 1890 and 1899 in a 36-volume edition in Paris (eds. A. and E. Borgnet). Since 1951 a new critical edition has been issued, which is still incomplete (Münster i.W., ed. B. Geyer).

Scientific methodology

When Albert wrote his paraphrases and commentaries on Aristotelian natural philosophy, it was his intention to give instruction to his students and confrères. Confronted with various contradictions and omissions in the work of *the philosopher*, Albert also relied on numerous other sources as well as on his own observations. In the area of medicine, *Galen* and *Avicenna* were his principle authorities, but he also read *Alhazen, Al-Farabi* and *Costa ben Luca* (*Constabulus*, 864–923), the Christian physician and philosopher from the Arabic world of Baalbek. Presumably Albert's circle in Cologne included several physicians with whom he appears to have discussed professional matters.[16] For Albertus Magnus medicine and natural philosophy shared a common ground and could well benefit from each other. There can be no doubt that Albert was seriously interested in empirical research. Although his understanding of the *experimentum* was not identical with that of the present day, he stated that experience has to be considered *not only in one way, but according to all circumstances*[17] in order to yield a correct research principle. He was also aware, however, that scientific activity often extends beyond what one can perceive with the sense organs:
"All our knowledge relates to and begins with perceptual experience. When, however, knowledge analyses the whole field of sensory experience, it does not deal only with the perceptual phenomena but transgresses those phenomena vehemently..."[18] Nevertheless Albert diligently collected literature his entire life as well as data and observations from his own experience which he considered to be of importance in understanding nature.

According to Albert the Great, natural sciences are not only independent of theology but also of mathematics; nevertheless logic and mathematics are *important tools in scientific research.* Albert disagreed with Grosseteste's view that the structure of the world follows simple general metaphysical principles and that mathematics holds an intermediate position between metaphysics and experience.[19] Albert also thought at length about how nature in its complexity could be the object of systematic reasoning. In giving an interpretation of Aristotle, he developed an 'asymmetric' model of a teleological interpretation of nature, allowing the scientist to draw conclusions from the effects back to the causes, but not vice versa, thereby denying any mechanistic determinism in nature.[20] It seems that in his interpretations goal-directed processes were the only means of overcoming the chaos of nature and understanding the structural and functional regularities appearing in plants and animals including man.

The soul and the brain in Albert's natural philosophy

Vision is the result of physiological processes in the eye and brain. It is therefore important to consider next the general principles assumed by Albert to characterize the function of the senses and the brain, and the psychophysical interaction related to their functions. The following delineation is based upon Albert's psychophysical theories of perception, as expounded in his *Summa de creaturis*, in *De anima* and in the *Parva naturalia*. Furthermore, his zoological opus *De animalibus* provides some clues to his knowledge of brain anatomy. Minor changes in his explanation of the brain-mind relation become evident in the course of time but are not taken into account here. Albert showed little respect for the theories of his Latin predecessors. Although he still believed in an immaterial and immortal *intellectus*, he tried to separate the speculative system of theology from empirical knowledge in his natural philosophy. The matter in which he treated this problem demonstrates the strong influence of Islamic Aristotelians, particularly from Avicenna, and also indicates his thorough knowledge of the Galenic tradition. Albert considered the soul as a functional entity, but he accepted the old Platonic division[21] into a vegetative, animal and rational soul. The *animal soul* included the powers of *sense perception*, its *central processing* and *reflectory or voluntary movements*. To Albert, there was no doubt that these faculties were closely linked to brain functions, as the doctrine of brain cell functions had been taught by some of the Hippocratic physicians and in particular by the *Alexandrinic school* of medicine (*Herophilos, Erasitratos*, 3rd century BC). Galen had propagated the cell doctrine and the Patristic theologians *Nemesios of Emesa* and *Aurelius Augustinus* had also accepted it for the interpretation of the mortal part of the soul (Fig. 2).

Albert believed that the nerves originating in the sense organs have their main endings in the frontal part of the brain. Presumably he was aware of the differences between the grey and white matter of the brain, which he described as consisting of a "*folded substance*", a "*medullary substance*" and

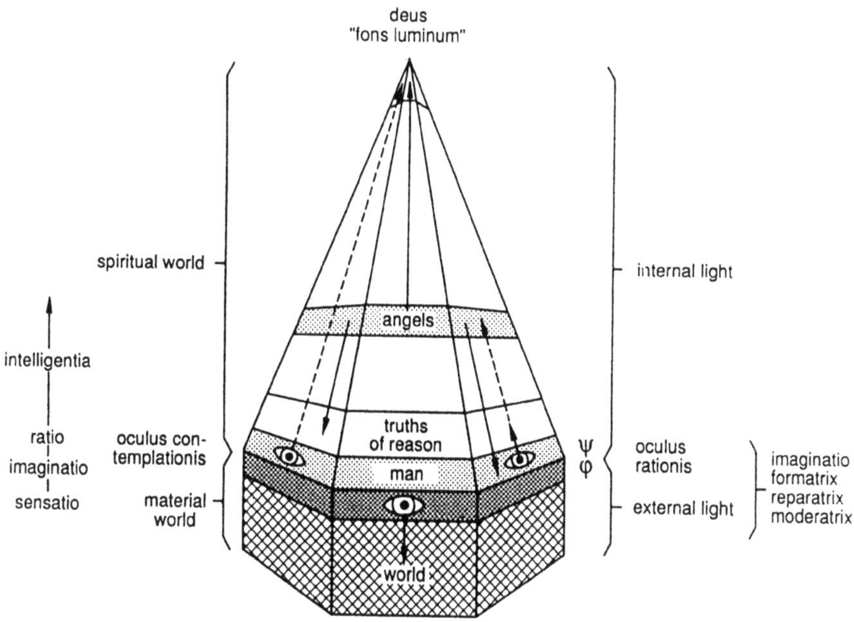

Fig. 1. Diagram of the ontological pyramid, the 'pyramid of spirit and light' representing the ideas of the Victorine theologians of the 12th century. Three classes of 'eyes' stand for different modes of experience and cognition. The *oculus carnis* represents the sense organs of the body, which receive signals from the material world. The *oculus rationis* is illuminated by internal light created by God and is directed towards the truths of reason, theological concepts or philosophical universals. It is capable of interacting with the angels positioned in the hierarchy of the pyramid between man and God. The *oculus contemplationis*, when illuminated sufficiently by light from the *fons luminum*, may experience God in the act of contemplation. The combination of information received by the *oculus carnis* and the *oculus rationis* endows man with cognitive abilities beyond the perception of the material world modifying, extending and creating new imaginations (*imaginatio moderatrix, reparatrix et formatrix*). For further explanation see text.

the "*ventricles*".[22] Central signal processing takes place within the *spiritus animalis*, which operates within the nerves and the ventricles, but also the brain substance along the inner surface of the three ventricles plays an important role. In regard to the function attributed to the heart, Albert encountered the traditional antagonism between Plato and Aristotle who disputed the location of the central organ of the soul (*hegemonikon*) as being either the brain (Plato) or the heart (Aristotle). Galen provided a sort of compromise between these views that was followed by Albert. As Galen he assumed that the *spiritus vitalis*, as the elementary type of spirit, is generated by distillation of blood within the heart, the hottest place in the body, and is transported through the arteries to the brain, where it is distilled into the *spiritus animalis* and refined to the *spiritus sensibilis* serving the sense organs and perception. The spirits' physical composition was believed to be between water and air, whereby every step of distillation made the spirit finer. Occasionally the spirit was also attributed properties of light.[23]

Albert's theory of vision

Since the days of the pre-Socratic philosophers vision had played an important role in demonstrating the importance of sensory function for cognition. Visual experience moreover was easily accessible to the self-observing scientist and provided many illusionary phenomena, illustrating the limits of sensory experience. Vision also depends on light, which played a venerable role in ancient cosmologies. Therefore many theories of vision are more than a mere description of a sense modality. This becomes especially evident when one regards the teachings of scholastic theologians on visual perception in the generations before Albert the Great.

Victorine predecessors in the 12th century. To demonstrate the progress in theories of vision achieved in the 13th century, we shall first give a brief outline of how sensory physiology had been integrated 100 years earlier into the general anthropological ideas of scholastic theology, which implemented Augustinian and Neoplatonic thinking to subordinate the sciences to a theological interpretation and to guarantee that philosophy and scientific thinking remained the *ancilla theologiae*, the handmaiden of theology. Knowledge of the world perceived through the senses was placed on the lowest level of the epistemological hierarchy. Cognition was believed to be only possible through *internal* and *external light*, which God as the fountain of light shed upon the world. The Creator first created light as the prime cosmological principle. From light the whole material cosmos and simultaneously the entire spiritual world developed. In the process of cognition light mediates the interaction within a hierarchical pyramid, from the top of which God as *fons luminum* sheds light on a number of angels located between Him and man, and on man himself placed at the lowest level of the pyramid.

The role of sense perception in such a model becomes apparent through the ideas of *Hugo of St. Victor* (ca 1096–1142) and his pupil, the Scot *Richard of St. Victor* (ca. 1115–1173).[24] Hugo, who probably stemmed from the family of the *Counts of Blankenburg*,[25] a small town on the eastern slopes of the Harz mountains in Germany, entered the abbey of St. Victor in Paris around the year 1115. He was the author of various theological writings, a systematic introduction to philosophy (*Didascalicon*)[26] and a psychological-philosophical treatise (*De unione corporis et animae*). He divided the sciences into four fields: theory, practice, mechanics and logic. Hugo and Richard illustrated the ability of man's cognition within the framework of a 'light pyramid' (Fig. 1) by means of three kinds of 'eyes' as a modification of the 'external' and 'internal' eyes of *Boethius* (about 480–524):[27] The *natural eye* [*oculus naturalis*] is a symbol for the senses and serves man in perception and understanding the structure of the everyday world. The rational eye [*oculus rationis*], in contrast, helps the soul to recognize itself and spiritual beings, accomplishing thereby the *divinitas*, theological knowledge. With the *mystic eye* [*oculus comtemplationis*] the soul can see God as the origin of all internal and external light and as the Creator of the material and spiritual world (Fig. 1).[28]

To Hugo and Richard of St. Victor as well as other scholastic theologians the limits of human knowledge were the consequence of the Fall of Man and the state of sin in which man is living. Man's rational and mystical eyes were blurred when he was driven out of paradise. This was not the case in the natural eyes, since we share them with the animals which cannot be guilty of any sin. This community of human and animal sense perception may have been the reason why Hugo in his theological system placed little weight on immediate experience. The sense organs, situated at a low level of experience within the theological hierarchy of cognition, however, were granted a certain degree of independence by the Victorine theologians. Perception with the natural sense organs available to man increases his knowledge and thus gives him access to the material world, as opposed to the angels who lack in sense organs. Angels have to communicate with mortal man within the light pyramid to obtain information about the material world. This interpretation would appear to indicate a touch of irony in scholastic theology.

Although Hugo and Richard of St. Victor were familiar with the Augustinian concepts and some of the Galenic tradition, they repeatedly emphasized that the soul of man was indivisible and not to be localized in a particular part of the body. Richard of St. Victor attributed a special function in perception and cognition to the head, with the argument that the head is placed at the top of the body as God is placed at the top of the light pyramid. Nevertheless, for the Victorine mystics it was superfluous to differentiate cognitive powers, as they were to be considered as functionally variable states of a uniform soul. It may come as no surprise therefore that Hugo of St. Victor did not really value medicine as an intellectual challenge and saw no need to include empirical data from the observations of physicians on brain lesions in his concept of man. In his view medicine belonged to the mechanical arts and was a "*suitable occupation for manually adept members of the lower classes*".[29]

Afferent and efferent mechanisms in perception. Discussing the principles of perception using vision as an example, Albert was confronted with the old theory that vision is only possible by the action of *efferent light* generated by the *spiritus sensibilis*, and *afferent light* generated by light sources in the extrapersonal space.[30] Plato had elaborated on the extramission theory of

Empedocles of Akragas, who believed that for the purpose of vision internal light leaves the eye, touches the objects and is reflected back to the lens of the eye where the primary physiological transduction occurs. Plato developed the concept that the internal light emitted through the pupil within a 'cone' or 'pyramid" interacts with the external light and forms the *body of vision*. This body of vision touches the objects, and the changes caused by these interactions are reflected back to the lens of the eye.[31] The order within the world of visual objects is maintained within the cone of vision. This was an early interpretation of the *visual field* of the eyes. Plato's *extramission theory* was rejected by Aristotle,[32] who considered the idea of efferent light leaving the eye to be just nonsense.

Albert settled for the Aristotelian viewpoint and assumed that perception is mainly a passive process, whereby the signals from the objects are transmitted by means of a *medium* to the sense organs. Affected by these signals the sense organs transmit their signals through the nerves to the *hegemonikon*, the central organ of the soul. Departing from Aristotle, and supporting the well-documented medical tradition, Albert considered the brain as the seat of the *hegemonikon*. In trying to understand how the senses dealt with the material percept, Albert used the term *species sensibilis* in reference to an example given by Aristotle. The latter had described how the form of a seal could be impressed on wax without any of its matter being transferred.[33] Such an *immaterial representation* of an object is what Albert meant by the *species sensibilis*. He believed that the *species* attains the sense organ through the *medium* where it is always potentially present. For the sense of vision water or air is an adequate *medium*. When trying to translate the term *species*, we found the modern word *signal* to be suitable – as long as the processes in the sensory systems are meant. The term *information* or *information content* seems to be a better expression when Albert talks about the *species* as contents of the perception (figs. 2, 3).

The interaction of the *species* and the sensible spirit within the sense organs constitutes the transduction process of the external signal into physiological events. This process ensures that only the form of the object without the matter is represented in the *spiritus sensibilis*. In the Galenic tradition the spiritus was considered a special substance in a gaseous state related to the 'elements' water and air. The spirits are subject to physical alterations, since their function depends on body temperature and their composition on the efficacy of certain distillation processes occurring between heart and brain and within the brain. Spiritus is found within the brain ventricle as well as in the nerves, which were believed to be hollow tubules. It not only serves as a medium for signal transport but may also be considered important in signal processing. Regarding the sense organs, the *spiritus sensibilis* flows in both directions. The *efferent spiritus flow* is present within the ventricle system (i.e. flow from the third brain cell – the fourth ventricle of modern anatomy – to the first brain cell, the lateral ventricles of modern anatomy), but also connects the first cell with the sense organs and the third brain cell with the muscles. The *afferent spiritus flow* originates within the sense organs and uses the sensory nerves by which the sense organs are connected with the brain, especially with the first cell. Under physiological conditions the spiritus flow was assumed to be 'smooth'. When the laminar spiritus flow was transformed into a turbulent flow, however, pathological symptoms would be the consequence.

Vision of the eye. Of the five senses known to Greek natural philosophers, traditionally the sense of vision was the sense modality scrutinized most closely. For Albert, it was the most significant sense in terms of recognizing and discerning the world, but in terms of mere survival vision seemed the least important, an opinion which followed traditional Aristotelian teaching. The power of vision is conducted through the optic nerve by the *spiritus visibilis* and resides in the crystalline humor, i.e. the lens of the eye. Only the *visible species* is able to cause the necessary alteration of the spirits in the eye, i.e. the specificity of sense perception lies in the organ of the senses.[34] Albert was convinced that in regard to elementary perception the senses do not err: "*The sense of vision will always indicate (the colour) red as red*".[35] Albert, however, considered any more complex judgements as potentially false. Concerning elementary mechanisms of vision, he was evidently not aware that the afterimage of a red flower seen on a white wall is green.

Albert's anatomical knowledge of the eye was comparable to that of the best-trained physicians of his time and encompassed almost all of the Arabic teachings extending Galen's physiology and pathophysiology of vision. In addition to the *crystalline humor*, the *lens*, which was believed to be located in the center of the eye, Albert discerned two more fluids:[36] the *vitreous humor* behind the lens and the *albuminous humor* (i.e. the aequous humor) shielding the front of the lens. Seven different 'membranes' envelop these fluids. The first is the retina in the rear part of the eye arising from the optic nerve, covering the internal surface. The most outer 'membrane' is the sheath of the 6 external eye muscles. Water was believed to be the prevailing element in the composition of the eye as it 'receives' forms easily and retains them better than air.[37] The importance of water in the eye becomes obvious when the tunics are injured either physically or by extensive 'heat' induced by strong light radiation or an overdose of alcohol. This was an empirical description of the main causes of a 'red eye'.

The detailed composition of the eye was also a major issue in the battle against the extramission theory. The exponents of this theory had postulated the existence of *fire* within the eye and referred to an old observation made by *Alcmaeon of Croton* (6th – 5th century BC): indentation of the eyeball leads to the perception of light, the *deformation phosphenes*.[38] As mentioned above, Albert rejected the extramission theory and took great pains to provide a different explanation of the deformation phosphenes, assuming that some of the *external light* received is retained in the eye and becomes visible in the case of deformation. Albertus Magnus also observed phosphenes appearing during rapid eye movements (saccades).[39] These 'saccadic phosphenes', already mentioned by Aristotle,[40] are caused by stretch of the retina around the papilla of the optic nerve during the rapid eye movements. Albert was correct in emphasizing that saccadic phosphenes can only be seen in complete darkness or with closed eyelids.[41] He gave a fairly detailed description on the perceived change in position of the saccadic phosphenes after each eye movement. When he moved his eyes quickly back and forth, Albert observed *two lights spots* simultaneously. This observation was correct.[42] The saccadic phosphene is evoked whenever a large saccade towards the midline is made. Since the stretch of the peripapillar retina outlasts the saccadic eye movements due to the plastic properties of the tissue, with rapid back and forth eye movements one can perceive simultaneously the saccadic phosphene evoked by stretch of the peripapillar retina in the left and right eye.

Albert's discussions on light generated within the eye were fairly cautious, however, and he left the question open whether some animals, especially those active at night, might emit *fiery particles* from their eyes. He also reported about *venomous serpents* and *menstruating women* which *infect* the air or the eyes of a casual spectator.[43] Without questioning the reliability of such observations, Albert did not admit them as arguments for the extramission theory, but explained them as *poisonous evaporations* which had nothing to do with sense perception.

The primary stimuli of vision are the *colours of the object surfaces* which become visible through light shining onto them.[44] According to Albert, light is neither a body nor does it consist of multiple light particles constantly emanating from a source or from the surface of visible objects, as Democritus and Epicurus had taught in their *eidola*-hypothesis.[45] Light is primarily the presence of a shining body in a transparent medium. It is transmitted with infinite velocity, i.e. *without time* through air and water[46] and propagates linearly. Albert used two terms for *light*: *lux* referred to the shining sources of light, *lumen* to the visible brightness of something being illuminated. The surface brightness makes the colours of the objects appear.[47] Chromaticity can occur in three ways: by coloured light emitted from a light source, by a coloured filter, i.e. coloured glass through which white light falls, or by coloured pigments of the surface of objects. Light, according to Albert, always generates heat and the colour of the light emitted depends on the mixture of 'warm' and 'cold' elements present in the light-emitting body, i.e. the temperature of the light source. With this remark Albert proved that he possessed a qualitative comprehension of the correlation between the temperature of a radiating body and its colour.[48]

In general, Albert made only limited use of Alhazen's *De aspectibus*[49] in his vision theory. He was in agreement, however, with most of Alhazen's ideas, e.g. the threshold of simultaneous perception of light sources of different intensities: one cannot see starlight or a glowworm during the daytime because their weak light is concealed by the much stronger light of the sun. Another remark of Alhazen also found Albert's approval: When speaking about the clearness of vision decreasing in the periphery of the visual field, he stated that one can only see what lies *in a straight line* to the eye. Albert elaborated on this explanation: "*It must be noted that all vision takes place in the form of a pyramid, whose base is on the visible object, and whose angle is at the center of the crystalline humor. Therefore, since the eye is at the apex, all the lines from the base of the pyramid to the angle are perpendicular to the eye and to the crystalline humor...*".[50] The lines constituting the pyramid must be considered as rectilinear alterations of the medium, and the strongest vision is along the line called *the axis of the pyramid*.[51] With this idea of a visual pyramid Albert also integrated Plato's concept of a *body of vision* or *visual cone*, as the great Greek opticians Euclid and Ptolemy called it. These ideas can be considered as an approach to a quantitative description of the *visual field of the eye*. By means of the visual rays within the pyramid of vision Albert also explained visual acuity: an object is only visible when its visual angle is larger than the minimum angle between the visual rays within the pyramid of vision.

Albert also explained *presbyopia* by means of the visual spirits acting within the eye and related to the cone of vision. Presbyopia in those days was a problem of the older scholars who had great difficulty reading their manuscripts. The systematic application of eye glasses or convex lens as 'reading stones' was still to come. Presbyopia, according to Albert, appears when "*the visual spirit is weakened as happens in the old and those who are dried out by wakefulness and study*".[52] Then the angle of the visual pyramid diminishes. When such persons want to see the entire object, they must hold it farther away from the eye. One realizes that this was a rather awkward interpretation of presbyopia, a better one becoming possible only after Johannes Kepler (1571–1630) had developed his theories on the visual optics of the eye and explained how a sharp inversed image is cast on the retinal surface.[53] On the other hand Albert must have had a vague idea of the inversed representation of the visual world within the eye, since he once argued that the eye operates as a *living convex mirror* and concluded from this fact that "*the right side of an object is located in the left part of the eye and vice versa*".[54] This remark, deduced from the observation of the first Purkyně image, is nevertheless still far removed from a realistic view of optical image formation in the eye.

Binocular vision and *double vision* were also topics treated by Albert. As the *visible forms leave their impressions in each of the two eyes*, he postulated a place within the brain, in agreement with Galen, where the species of the two eyes could unite adequately to render binocular vision. Traditionally this duty was assigned to the chiasm of the optic nerves and Albert followed the Galenic tradition in this respect. He was aware, however, that binocular fusion could be disturbed and listed various reasons *why one thing is seen as two*.[55] He thought that most of the disturbances in binocular fusion can be attributed to a dysfunction occurring at the intersection of the two optic nerves in the chiasm. Sometimes it just 'happens' that one of the nerves is detached from the point of contact, thereby impeding a combination of the forms received by the two eyes. This occurs, for example, when one displaces one eye in its orbit by slight pressure of the finger. Double vision can also be caused, however, *by irregularities in the flow of the visual spirit.* When this flow is disturbed, the visual spirits do not receive the species of each eye in the necessary order to combine them with each other. Such a condition appears when the visual spirit leaves its natural space, i.e., the hollow optic nerve. But even when the visual spirit remains within the nerve canals, problems in binocular fusion may arise when the efferent and afferent flow of the *spiritus visibilis* disturb each other. Albert assumed this to be the case when too much wine consumption leads to an "*excessive heat*" of the visual spirits. Since temperature differences were traditionally believed to be the driving force of the spiritus movement within the brain and the sense organs, the assumption that 'excessive heat' transforms laminar into turbulent spiritus flow and thus leads to perceptual disturbances was in those days a plausible explanation of double vision. A turbulent flow of the spiritus visibilis was also believed to be the cause of the involuntary eye movements (nystagmus) observed by Albert in alcoholics. Similarly, impairment in visual perception after extended vestibular stimulation (e.g., a long boat journey) was explained by a disturbance in the flow of the *spiritus visibilis*.[56]

Albert observed that an *unnatural widening or narrowing* of the pupils could result in misjudgment of object size. He evidently meant reports on micropsia or macropsia from patients who suffered from inadequate control of vergence and/or accommodation.

Based on the publications of later generations on the structure of the optic chiasm, it is highly probable that the anatomy of Albert the Great's time believed that the optic nerves only touch each other at the optic chiasm and remain on the side *ipsilateral* to the eye of origin on their way to the brain. Albert, however, seemed to have modified this idea. He reported on a soldier who had been wounded in the left temple and lost his vision in the *right eye*.[57] It is not clear whether Albert examined him personally, but it seems rather probable that *right eye* and the *right half of the visual fields of both eyes* were mixed up. Albert's observation, however, forced him to conclude that the optic nerve fibers cross totally to the other side of the brain: "*... a soldier who was wounded in the left temple, lost vision of his right eye, which certainly happened because of the crossing of the nerves directed from the eyes to the front of the head, as we have said above...*"[58]

In the same paragraph Albert discusséd the observation that following traumatic lesions of the optic nerve, vision does not return. He thought that "*because of the hardness of the scar the passage through which light carried from the crystalline (humor) of the eye by which the spirit must travel, is blocked, and thus there is darkness as when a lamp is extinguished.*"[59]

Albert's discussion on vision and optics of the eye touched upon numerous other subjects: he attempted to develop a systematic theory on the mutual relations of perceived colours and considered some of them to be *symmetric* since they seemed to display a certain proportion to each other. Every colour is attributed to a certain species for which the opposite also exists (e.g., black-white). This statement may be interpreted as an early version of the theory of colour opponency ('Gegenfarbentheorie') as developed in the 19th century by *Ernst Mach* and *Ewald Hering*. '*Symmetric contrasts*' are '*delectabilis*' to the observer.[60] Moreover, Albert clearly recognized that vision is based on two perceptual categories depending on the average luminance of a visual scene or on light-dark adaptation respectively. Thus he discerned between the ability to see colours and to distinguish between bright and dark: "*In the bright, vision perceives the coloured, whereas in the dark, it perceives the bright*".[61] This was a clear description of the phenomenological principles of the modern *duplicity theory*, i.e., the well-supported assumption that colour vision is cone vision under photopic conditions of daylight, while achromatic scotopic vision operates under the conditions of moon- and starlight illumination and is mediated by the rods of the retina. Albert also mentioned people who are unable to see under daylight conditions but succeed fairly well by moonlight: He had evidently observed a rod monochromat.[62] *Short-sightedness* he attributed to a 'dislocation' of the crystalline lens towards the rear part of the eye.[63] Finally he discussed light reflection on smooth surfaces and treated the phenomena of transient dazzling as well as visual afterimages.

Albert's genuine interest in anything connected with vision is evident. On his long trips his eyes were his most important sense organ in gathering substantial empirical material, which he tried to integrate into his general theory of nature. Thus it is not surprising that he dealt a great deal with vision and its anatomical and physiological conditions.

The central processing of the sense data; steps from perception to cognition

In the following, Albert's theory of cognition is presented. This theory followed closely the Arabic tradition, especially the concepts of *Avicenna, Costa ben Luca* and *Alhazen* and, of course, also included object perception and recognition by means of vision. Albert's model of the different cerebral processes is an extension of earlier models discussed by Patristic theologians who had adapted Galen's concepts on this matter. Albert also gained knowledge of the Galenic tradition through *Nemesios of Emesa* (flourished 390 – 400 AD), whom he quoted as *Gregor of Nyssa*. Fig. 2 illustrates the principles of cognitive functions described by Nemesios in his book *De natura hominis*.[64] Three different 'internal forces, *sensus communis, cognitio* and *memoria*', are housed in the three brain cells. The afferent and efferent

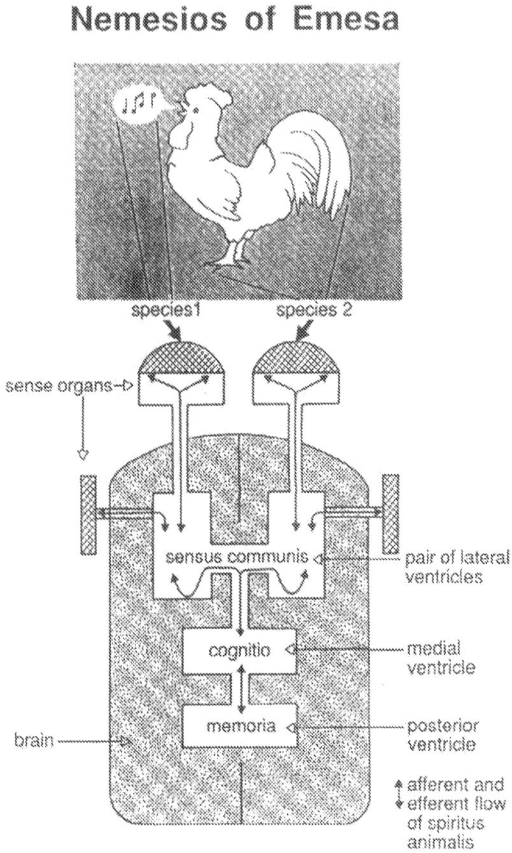

Fig. 2. Schematic representation of the Galenic model of elementary cognitive functions and their location in the cerebral ventricles. The figure represents the description of Nemesios of Emesa. For further explanation see text (From Grüsser, 1990, modified).

spiritus flow between the sense organs and the first brain cell mediates the perceptual mechanisms; the spiritus flow between the first and third brain cells organises the cognitive functions. Albert elaborated on this model, which was also accepted with some modification by Aurelius Augustinus,[65] and, under the influence of Avicenna and Alhazen, proposed the concept illustrated in Fig. 3 and discussed in the following.[66]

The common sense (sensus communis). According to Albert all sense organs are connected by hollow nerves with the frontal part of the brain, in particular the first brain. When Albert spoke about the first brain cell he clearly knew that it consists of two parts, i.e., the two lateral ventricles.[67] Within the *anterior part* of this cavity arrive all signals transported by the *spiritus sensibilis* from the sense organs of the five external senses. The

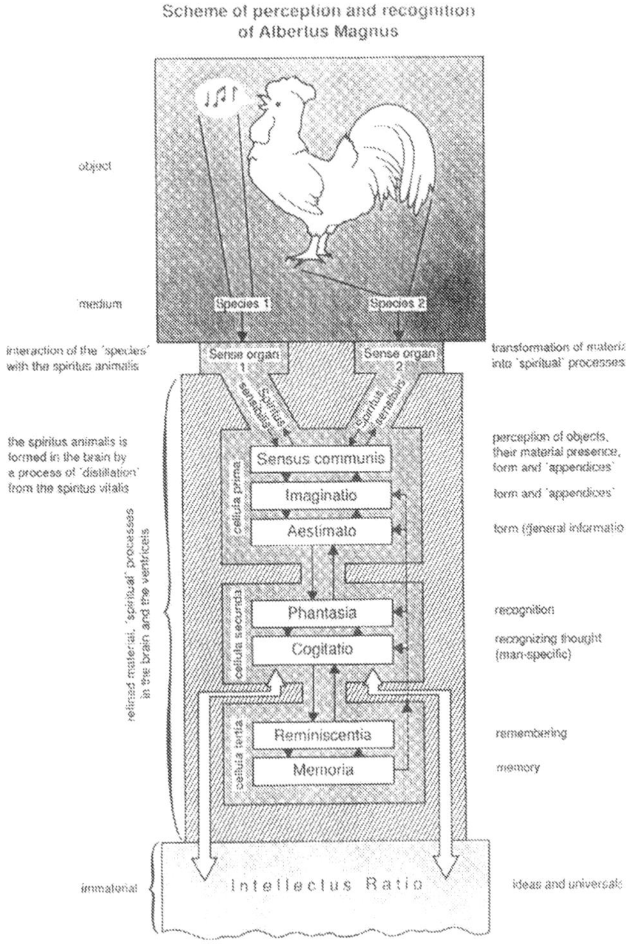

Fig. 3. Schematic representation of the scheme of perception, recognition and cognition of Albertus Magnus. For further explanation see text (from Grüsser, 1990, modified).

sensus communis, residing in this anterior section of the first brain cavity, was considered to be the first of the *internal powers*.[68] The common sense as the *fountain of senses* integrates the sensory signals and links the results of this integration to the other internal powers.

In Albert's model, multimodal integration occurring in the *sensus communis* has various aspects: Firstly it is attributed the function ascribed today to the cortical association areas: to judge that an object is both white and sweet simultaneously. However the common sense can also combine signals referring not only to the same object but also to one and the same property of an object, for example when one perceives through either vision or touch that the surface of a body is rough. Finally spatio-temporal integration also belongs to the duties of the *sensus communis*: Albert used the example of the phonetic sequence of human speech revealing its meaning only when it is merged into characteristic syllables, words and sentences of a distinct language. Based on these spatio-temporal integration functions the common sense judges the five general qualities of the perceived objects: *size, shape, quantity, motion* and *permanence*.

The *sensus communis* is not only a function integrating afferent sense signals but also the mechanism controlling the efferent flow of the *spiritus sensibilis*. By regulating the quantity of efferent spiritus flow the common sense can diminish or augment the sensitivity of any sense organ. The *sensus communis* transmits the *intentio animae*. With respect to vision, Albert wrote: "*The intention facilitates the outflow of the spiritus sensibilis similarly as an increase in temperature opens the pores*" [of the skin?].[69] The sensus communis 'distributes' the spiritus sensibilis to the different sense organs.[70] Assuming that the overall efficacy, the thresholds and the operative precision of the sense organs are under the control of efferent spiritus flow, Albert designed a physiological model of *general and spatially directed attention*. Although Albert refuted all theories of *internal light* as postulated by the Victorine mystics or by Robert Grosseteste, he was nevertheless influenced by their views. Once he mentioned that light was responsible for the spiritual representation of all perceived objects.[71] What he wanted to express was probably the high degree of similarity he assumed to exist between light and the *spiritus animalis*, since he considered the latter to be a *lucid and subtle substance*[72] produced from the more material *spiritus naturalis* (see above).

The *sensus communis* only provides the basic level of abstraction. Its function is of necessity bound to the maintained presence of the perceived objects: "*Being a sense, it receives the species of the objects without matter, yet in the presence of matter*".[73] On the other hand, a somewhat higher degree of abstraction was also attributed to the *sensus communis*, since Albert believed that through the common sense we become conscious of our own sensing by noticing that we hear, see, touch etc.[74] Thus the *sensus communis* plays a double role: it is the highest level of elementary sensory perception by the outer senses, the *vis apprehensiva deforis*, and simultaneously the doorway to the inner senses, the *vis apprehensiva deintus*.[75]

Imagination. Further afferent signal flow within the brain cells contributes to the next steps of cognition. During the flow of the *spiritus animalis* through the three ventricles from the anterior part of the brain to the occipital part, the refinement of the spiritus sensibilis parallels increase in degree of abstraction in the cognitive process. Located in the first cerebral cell immediately to the rear of the *sensus communis*, the *imaginatio* retains the species of the perceived object even when the object has disappeared from the perceived extrapersonal space. This independence of the *imaginatio* from the presence of objects affecting the sense organs is achieved by a short-term memory and marks the second level of abstraction.[76] The preserved *imago* of the perceived object still displays accidental and contingent properties like the colour of the face or the shape of a person just observed. Acting longer than the sense stimulus, the *imaginatio* has much in common with the present-day *iconic memory* of vision[77] and those brief visual after-effects attributed mainly to cerebral neuronal mechanisms.

Although Albert left no doubt that the internal senses are physiological functions based on material structures, he varied in his interpretations of the role of the spiritus animalis and the brain substance in cognition. In *De anima* he closely followed Avicenna, stating that the perceived forms had their cerebral representations corresponding in shape, size and position.[78] With these remarks Albert presumably favoured the idea of *linear representation* of the perceived world within the brain. This idea was later pursued by *Leonardo da Vinci*,[79] who believed that the walls of the cerebral ventricles serve as a projection plane of the cerebral mechanisms responsible for the visual percept.

Estimation, phantasy and cognition. The internal powers *estimatio, phantasia* and *cognitio* elaborate on the further abstraction of the percept to reach the highest level in the process of cognition. Since their functions are closely mingled, Albert localized these three powers jointly in the rear of the first and in the second ventricles (Fig. 3).[80] The power of estimation is able to "*elicit the intentions*"[81] which are not directly depicted in the sense data, yet would never come to our attention without sense perception. Thus, estimatio can reach a judgement upon something as being pleasant or unpleasant. It was believed to be an *instinctive power* – Albert indeed used the term 'instinct'. *Estimatio* provides the decision whether the object should be approached or avoided. While animals inevitably follow the same innate pattern of behaviour, like the sheep always fleeing from the wolf without having ever seen it, human beings are able to use and generalize their sensory experiences and integrate them into the function of *estimatio* for later decisions based on sense data.[82] With this concept Albert pursued ideas akin to the modern *inborn release mechanisms* triggered by biologically relevant *key stimuli.* This concept was repeatedly discussed towards the end of the 19th century by *Ernst Mach*[83] and *Ewald Hering*[84] and integrated during the last generation by *Lorenz, Tinbergen* and their pupils into a reasonable model of instinctive behaviour.[85] As Albert correctly recognized, it is evident that even *elementary inborn releasing mechanisms* are modified by experience.[86]

Phantasia is an internal faculty possessed by all higher animals. It is of a highly integrative power and creates the *phantasma* by "*composing the images with the intentions, the images with the images and the intentions with the intentions for a twofold purpose*".[87] The first of the operations of *phantasia* is of a cognitive nature: we recognize someone as a human being, independent of his or her actual appearance. The second property aims at some behavioural consequence in man and animals: Albert used the example of animals collecting and 'storing' food for lengthy periods or building their home in a sophisticated manner. Finally in analogy to *estimatio, phantasia* was attributed the ability to judge a fact as being true or false.

As mentioned above, of all living beings only man was believed to participate in the immateral *intellect* by means of his *rational soul.* In Albert's model *phantasia* plays a prominent role in this dualistic view. *Phantasia* has developed in man into *cognitio*, a power which only man possesses. The physiological mechanisms of *cognitio* and *phantasia* served in Albert's model as *relays* by which the immortal soul interacts with the material processes.[88] Albert once wrote: "*Haec [phantasia] etiam est illa quae intellectualia assimilat corporalibus*".[89] Thus the physiological processes of *phantasia* and *cognitio* serve functionally the same purpose as Descartes attributed to the pineal organ or Eccles to the "*open modules*" of cortical neuronal networks.[90] The postulate of such a relay mechanism is a necessary requirement of all dualistic models of cognition when the partisans of dualism try to adapt neurological knowledge on cognitive brain functions and their impairment by brain lesions to their brain-mind models.

Albert was aware of the necessity of finding a distinct part of the brain where the immortal soul interacts with material processes. He considered a place which was different in the human brain in his opinion than in the brain of brutes.[91] In man, the *cognitive* or *syllogistic* portion of *phantasia* was located by him in the second brain cavity. This cavity – the third ventricle of modern anatomy – was described by Albert as a small passage for the *spiritus animalis*. Here he believed the animal spirit to be the most subtle and thus apt to activate the most complex brain functions as a relay of *cognitio* with the immortal *intellectus*.

Memory and reminiscence. While the internal powers described in the preceding were the subject of many disputes among medieval scientists and physicians, a general agreement existed on the delineation of the storing faculties of the memory and the function of reminiscence as discussed in the psychology of Plato and Aristotle. As proposed in the early brain cell model of Galen (Fig. 2), Albert located *memoria* and *reminiscentia* in the third brain cell, i.e., the fourth ventricle of present-day anatomy, where the powers for *voluntary and reflectory movements* also reside and act through the *spiritus animalis* descending from the occiput into six motor nerves (Fig. 3). Albert argued for this localization by quoting reports of patients with brain injuries in corresponding sites.

Organic mnemonic functions have two aspects: memory and reminiscence, storage and reactivation. *Memoria* stores what has been perceived by the external senses and is then assimilated by the internal senses. This storage also always contains a marker on the time the respective event occurred. *Memoria* differs from the short-term retentive functions performed by the *imaginatio*. In man, however, memoria also *accidentally* stores the *phantasma* developed after the interaction of sense data with the immaterial intellect.[92] Thus, *universal principles* drawn from experience also find their way into a material engram in the brain as do thoughts.

Reminiscentia describes the process of remembering something that has sunk into oblivion. Being a brain function specific to man, it commences with an act of the rational soul and follows the principles of custom, necessity and probability on its path to recollection. Reminiscentia organizes four components: it is an *act of rational decision* which begins from a *certain content* of actualized memory and has a *certain object as its goal*. Hereby the object of reminiscentia is related to a *certain event* in the past.[93] Since *reminiscentia* is an organic brain power, it may fall victim to detrimental influences like those appearing in the process of aging. The material process of memory difficulties appearing in aging man was explained by Albert as a decrease in the *humidity* of the brain which occurred in parallel to a general change in the physical *complexion*.[94] Thus the loss of memory and recollection observed in aging persons was not attributed in those days to a dysfunction of the *spiritus animalis* but to a change in the imprintability of the brain substance. It seems probable that some of the people reaching old age during Albert's time also suffered from Alzheimer's disease or other cerebral causes of memory dysfunction. It is reported that in the last year of his life Albert himself had to struggle with the typical loss of memory he had described earlier in his books.

The immaterial aspects of the soul. When the human intellect as part of the rational soul 'illuminates' the internal powers of *phantasia* or *cognitio*, the highest level of abstraction may be attained. Independent of all physical conditions, the intellect then elicits the essence (*quidditas*) of sense perceptions.[95] In complex metaphysical argumentations Albert succeeded in reconciling the Aristotelian theory with Christian dogma, granting individual immortality to human beings,[96] which was denied by some of the Arabic Aristotelians. Like Thomas Aquinas, who moulded much of Albert's thinking into a more orthodox doctrine, Albert refuted the concept of *innate universal* ideas. Dualism, however, was never questioned; it possessed such a high degree of plausibility in Western philosophy and theology that neither Albert nor Thomas Aquinas doubted this basic concept or spent much time thinking about the mode of transition from the material to the immaterial world, once the cerebral psychophysical relay structures had been defined.

Sleep and dreams

In discussing sleep and dreams Albert demonstrated how his psychophysical model of brain function was to be applied. Following the Arabic interpretation of Aristotle,[97] Albert developed a fairly mechanistic explanation of sleep: it occurs when the animal spirits are cooled down and *cold* dominates in the brain. As the vapors ascending to the brain condense, they obstruct the hollow nerves at the site where they leave the brain cells. Thus the normal flow of the *spiritus animalis* is blocked during sleep and voluntary movements and outer sense perception become impossible.[98] During sleep the spiritus visibilis retract from the eye. Therefore one does not see when the eyes are opened during sleep.[99] The internal brain functions, however, adapt to the cold and continue to operate since cooling is a part of their natural condition. At this stage the main flow of the spiritus animalis through the brain chambers reverses: "*Somnium est factum per reversionem evaporationis tenuis et lucidae..*".[100] i.e., the efferent spiritus flow from the third to the second and the second to the first brain cell dominates. When one dreams many little pictures are dissolved from *phantasia* and transported by the *spiritus animalis* in an efferent direction to the common sense, where they are regarded as true sense perceptions. Albert, however, was cautious in attributing *all* dreams to this physiological mechanism. He still accepted the possibility that some dreams may disclose a symbolic or prophetic meaning and have their origins beyond organic causes or changes in brain function.

Neuropsychiatric disorders

The brain function model of Albert the Great contained two mechanisms which could be disturbed by pathological processes: the operation and flow of the *spiritus animalis* within the sense organs, the cerebral ventricles and nerves, and the structure and function of the brain substance located around the ventricles. Albert explained *epileptic seizures* as resulting from *abundant humors* rising from the body into the brain and affecting the transport of the *spiritus animalis* through the nerves. He postulated a similarity between the effect of pathophysiological mechanisms leading to epilepsia and that leading to dreams since he was aware that epileptic seizures often occur during sleep and can then be particularly dangerous to life.[101] Albert was also conscious of the detrimental effects of excessive and chronic alcohol consumption on brain function and explained the changes in the brain of an alcoholic by the production of excessive amounts of *spiritus animalis* which is released from the brain and threatens to enlarge the veins of the throat, thus causing suffocation.

From literature and most likely from his own observations, Albert was acquainted with the state of *melancholia*, a nomenclature of the traditional medicine comprising various psychopathological conditions which in contemporary psychiatry are attributed to different diagnostic categories.[102] Following the Galenic tradition Albert believed that an excess of *black bile* modifies the physical and psychological constitution of man and leads to depression and acute psychotic disorders. He knew that patients suffering from 'melancholia' often sleep fitfully, have violent or dreadful dreams and alter their eating habits. Even when consuming large amounts, some still believe they will soon die of starvation. In Albert's opinion these patients suffer from an excess of *phantasia* but also seem to be predisposed to *amentia*.

Psychotic hallucinations were explained by Albert in a similar fashion as dreams, namely as being caused by a reversed spiritus flow (see above). He also believed the same abnormality to cause *logorrhoea, stereotyped* and *repeated phrases, abnormal singing* and other psychotic symptoms like obsessive remembering of the past. These states indicate uncontrollable involuntary actions induced by an activation of part of the memory stores during *reminiscentia*.[103] Albert discussed some external causes of psychotic states such as sensory deprivation, physical illness accompanied by high fever and exhaustive mental and intellectual effort, which were all believed to sometimes lead to hallucinations and loss of reality. Heautoscopy (i.e., seeing one's own double) was explained by Albert as a kind of visual mirror effect occurring in dense and humid air[104] and was not attributed to pathological cerebral processes.

These short descriptions of Albert's ideas on psychiatry indicate that he was willing to apply his quasi-mechanistic brain function model as a tool to understanding different symptoms appearing in acute or chronic psychoses. There is no indication that he supported superstitions explaining psychotic states as obsession by the devil or evil spirits, despite the fact that in later generations texts attributed to Albert were used by clerics and others for magical practice and sorcery.

Acknowledgement

The work was begun 1988/89 while the senior author (O.–J.G.) was supported by an Akademie-Stipendium of the *Stiftung Volkswagenwerk*. P.Th. was supported by a Nafög-fellowship of the Freie Universität Berlin. We thank Mrs J. Dames for her expert help in the English translation, Mrs B. Krawczynski and Mrs D. Starke for the art work and Mrs U. Saykam for typing the manuscript, which is an extended version of a talk presented at the meeting of the Hirschberg Society at Dresden, 26 October 1991 (Grüsser and Theiss, 1992).

Notes

1. Grabmann 1926, Vol.2, p. 325.
2. *De anima*, cf. Flasch 1986, p. 321.
3. Ashley 1980, p. 74.
4. McEvoy 1982.
5. Russell 1945, p. 463 ff.
6. Thorndike 1929; Leirtz 1948; Crombie 1953; Lindberg 1983.

7. See Craemer-Ruegenberg 1980; Dirrigl 1980; Layer 1980; Scheeben 1980; Weisheipl 1980b; Eckert 1981.
8. Balss 1947.
9. Schipperges 1980.
10. Flasch 1986, p. 246 ff.; McEvoy 1982.
11. Bach 1881; Bonné 1935.
12. Haubst 1952, 1980; Meuthen 1964.
13. A German translation of *De anima* is available in Theiss 1993.
14. Paradiso X.
15. Super Dionysium. De divinis nomibus (ed. Col) T. 37, p. 2, 51–56; Fries 1981.
16. Siraisi 1980, p. 390.
17. *Ethica*, VI, tr. 2, c. 25.
18. *De anima* T7, p. 2, 52–3,5.
19. Baur 1917; Wallace 1980b, p. 389.
20. Wallace 1980a, p. 114 ff.
21. Plato, *Timaios*.
22. *De animalibus* I, t. 3, c. 1 (ed. Stadler).
23. See below.
24. Ebner, 1917.
25. Derlingius 1745; Taylor 1957.
26. English translation Taylor 1961.
27. *Consolatio philosophiae* [*Trost der Philosophie*], I.V pros. 4.
28. Cf. also Ebner 1917; Ostler 1906; Schlette 1961.
29. Siraisi 1980, p. 383.
30. On the history of the extramission theories see Grüsser 1986.
31. Plato *Timaios*, cf. figs. 2 and 3 in Grüsser and Hagner 1990.
32. Theophrast *Peri aisthesis*, Stratton 1917.
33. Aristotle, *De anima*, 424 a.
34. *Summa de homine* (in *Summa de creaturis*), Quaestio XXXIV, p. 317 (ed. Borgnet).
35. *Ibid.*, p. 299.
36. *Ibid*, Quaestio XIX, p. 93.
37. *De sensu et sensato*, cap. 13, p. 178 (ed. Akdogan 1978).
38. Albert described deformation phosphenes in *Summa de creaturis*, Quaestio XX, 11, p. 169 (ed. Borgnet); On the history of deformation phosphenes see Grüsser 1986, Hagner 1987 and Grüsser and Hagner 1990.
39. *De sensu et sensato*, cap 4, p. 109 (ed. Akdogan).
40. *Ibid*, 437b.
41. *Ibid*, cap. 3, p. 105.
42. *Ibid*, cap. 4, p. 109.
43. *De anima*, lib. 2, tr. 3, cap. 1, p. 97 ff. (ed. Col).
44. *Ibid*, lib 2, tr. 3, cap. 7, p. 108.
45. Diels, Kranz 1951, II, p. 81 ff; Theophrast of Eresos, Stratton 1917, p. 109 ff.
46. *Summa de homine*, Quaestio XXI, Art. IV.
47. *Ibid*, Quaestio XXI, Art. II.
48. According to Planck's radiation law and the wave-length shift with temperature ('Wien's shift') the wave-lengths of the light emitted by a radiating dark body depend on the absolute temperature (degrees Kelvin) of that body.
49. Lindbert 1987, p. 194.
50. *De sensu et sensato*, cap. 14, p. 195 (ed. Akdogan).
51. *Ibid*, p. 187.
52. *Ibid*, p. 185.
53. Kepler *Ad Vitelloni paralipomena* 1604; *Dioptrice* 1611.
54. *De anima*, lib.2, tr. 3, cap. 14.
55. *De sensu et sensato*, cap. 11, p. 167–170 (the entire chapter is devoted to this question).

56. *De anima*, lib. 2, tr. 3, cap. 14.
57. *De sensu et sensato* (transl. by Akdogan 1978), cap. 14, p. 183.
58. *Ibid*, cap. 14. p. 182 ff.
59. *Ibid*, p. 192.
60. *Summa de homine*, Vol. II, Quaestio XXI, p. 196.
61. *De anima*, lib. 2, tr. 3, cap. 7.
62. *Ibid*, lib. 2, tr. 3, cap. 14.
63. *De sensu et sensato*, cap. 14, p. 184. It is probable that Albert believed (as Roger Bacon) that the lens is normally placed in the centre of the eyeball.
64. Telfer 1955; Verbeke, Moncho 1975. Galen's ideas are discussed in Hirschberg 1899/1912.
65. De Gen. Lit VII, 18.
66. Domanski 1900; Leyhdecker 1927; Wolfson 1935; Gasson 1963; Steneck 1970, 1980; Harvey 1975.
67. *De animalibus*, lib. 12, tr. 2, cap. 4, p. 849.
68. *De anima*, lib. 2, tr. 4, cap. 7, p. 156.
69. *Summa de creaturis* Quaestio XXI, Art. V, p. 209 (ed. Borgnet).
70. *Ibid*, Quaestio XXXV, Art. II, p. 313.
71. *De anima*, lib. 2, tr. 3, cap. 6, p. 105.
72. *De somno et vigilia*, lib. 1, tr. 1, cap. 7, p. 131 ff.
73. *De animalibus*, lib. 2, tr. 4, cap. 7, p. 156.
74. *Ibid*, lib. 2, tr. 4, cap. 8, p. 158.
75. Cf. also Arnold 1963; Harvey 1975.
76. *Ibid*, lib. 3, tr. 1, cap. 1, p. 167.
77. Sperling 1967.
78. *De animalibus*, lib. 3, tr. 1, cap. 4, p. 169ff. – For a discussion on the contradiction between *De anima* and the *Summa de homine* see Schneider 1903. p. 157ff.
79. Grüsser, 1990.
80. For a detailed discussion on localization and classification see Steneck, 1974.
81. *De anima*, lib. 3, tr. 1, cap. 2, p. 167.
82. *Ibid*, lib. 3, tr. 1, cap. 2, p. 168.
83. Mach 1885/1906.
84. Hering 1870/1912.
85. Cf. Eibl-Eibesfeldt 1970.
86. Grüsser, Grüsser-Cornehls 1968.
87. *De anima* lib. 3, tr. 1, cap. 3, p. 168.
88. *Ibid*, lib. 2, tr. 4, cap. 7, p. 157 and *Summa de homine*, II, Quaestio XXXVIII, p. 331.
89. *De anima*, lib. 2, tr. 4, cap. 7, p. 157, 97–98.
90. Descartes, *De homine* 1664; Popper and Eccles, *The self and its brain* 1977; Eccles 1986, 1990.
91. Steneck, 1974, p. 204 ff.
92. *Liber de memoria et reminescentia*. tr. 1, cap. 3, p. 103 (ed. Borgnet).
93. *Summa de creaturis*, Quaestio XXXXI, p. 352 (ed. Borgnet); cf. also Arnold 1963.
94. *Liber de memoria et reminiscentia*, tr. 2, cap. 7, p. 117 f.
95. *De anima*, lib. 2, tr. 3, cap. 5, p. 502.
96. For a more complete discourse see Bonné 1935; Dähnert 1934; Ogarek 1931; Reylly 1934; Schneider 1903.
97. Schneider, 1903, p. 142 ff.
98. *De somno et vigilia*, lib. 1, tr. 2, cap. 9. p. 152 (ed. Borgnet).
99. *Summa de creaturis* Quaestio XX, p. 170ff. (ed. Borgnet).
100. *De somno et vigilia*, lib. 2, tr. 1, cap. 4, p. 163.
101. *Ibid*, lib. 1, tr. 2, cap. 8, p. 150 f. Modern neurology discriminates between three types of sleep-related seizures: those occurring when the patient falls asleep, those appearing during the state of deep sleep with synchronized slow waves in the electroencephalogram and those fits triggered by the process of awakening (Janz 1969).

102. Cf. Kopp 1933, p. 58; Schmidt-Degenhard 1990; DSM 3-R classification. American Psychiatric Association, Spitzer and Williams 1987.
103. *De memoria et reminiscentia*, tr. 2, cap. 7, p. 118.
104. *De anima*, lib. 2. tr. 2, cap. 15.

References

Akdogan C. (1978). Optics in Albert the Great's 'De sensu et sensato': An Edition, English Translation, and Analysis. Diss., Wisconsin-Madison, 267 p.

Aristoteles (1983). Von der Seele. In: O. Gigon, ed. and transl. Vom Himmel/Von der Seele/Von der Dichtkunst. München: Deutscher Taschenbuch Verlag. pp. 181–347.

Aristoteles (1957). Parva Naturalia: On dreams. Text and translation in Aristotle Works. Vol. 7. London: Heinemann, pp. 348–371.

Arnold M.B. (1963). The internal senses: Functions or powers?, Part 2. The Thomist 26:15–34.

Ashley B.M. (1980). St. Albert and the nature of natural science. In: J. Weisheipl, ed., Albertus Magnus and the Sciences. Commemorative Essays. Toronto: Pontifical Institute of Mediaeval Studies, pp. 73–102.

Bach J. (1881). Des Albertus Magnus Verhältnis zu der Erkenntnisslehre der Griechen, Lateiner, Araber und Juden. Ein Beitrag zur Geschichte der Noetik. Wien. Reprint: Frankfurt a.M.: Minerva, 1966, 212 p.

Balss H. (1947). Albertus Magnus als Biologe: Werk und Ursprung. Stuttgart.

Baur L. (1917). Die Philosophie des Robert Grosseteste, Bischof von Lincoln. Münster i.W.: Aschendorff, 298 p.

Boethius A.M.T.S. (1990). Trost der Philosophie. (Consolatio philosophiae] E. Gegenschatz and O. Gigon, eds. München: Artemis. 369p.

Bonné J. (1935). Die Erkenntnislehre Alberts des Grossen mit besonderer Berücksichtigung des arabischen Neuplatonismus. Phil. Diss., Bonn 67p.

Costa ben Luca (1878). De differentia animae et spiritus. In: C. Barach, ed. Bibliotheca Philosophorum Mediae Aetatis. Innsbruck: Wagner'schen Universitäts-Buchhandlung, 2:120–139.

Craemer-Ruegenberg I. (1980). Albertus Magnus. München: Beck, 188p.

Crombie A.C. (1953). Robert Grosseteste and the origins of experimental science. Oxford: Charendon Press, 369p.

Dähnert U. (1934). Die Erkenntnislehre des Albertus Magnus, gemessen an den Stufen der 'Abstractio'. In: W. Schingnitz, ed., Studien und Bibliographien zur Gegenwartsphilosophie, Vol. 4, Leipzig: S. Hirzel, 277p.

Derlingius Ch.G. (1745). Dissertatio historica de Hugo S. Victore Comite Blankenburgensis. Helmstedt: Weygand, 32p.

Descartes R. (1664), De homine. In: K.E. Rothschuh, ed. (1969), R. Descartes. Über den Menschen (1632) sowie Beschreibung des menschlichen Körpers (1648).

Diels K. and Kranz W. (1951). Die Fragmente der Vorsokratiker. Griechisch und Deutsch. Basel: Weidmann, 3 Vols.

Dirrigl M. (1980). Albertus Magnus: Bischof von Regensburg, Theologe, Philosoph und Naturforscher. Regensburg: Buchverlag der Mittelbayerischen Zeitung, 111p.

Domanski B. (1900). Die Psychologie des Nemesios. Münster i.W.: Aschendorff, 168 p.

Ebner J. (1917). Die Erkenntnislehre Richards von St. Viktor. Münster i.W.: Aschendorff, 126p.

Eccles J.C. (1986). Do mental events cause neural events analogously to the probability fields of quantum mechanics?, Proc Roy Soc Lond B 227: 407–428.

Eccles J.C. (1990). Gehirn und Seele: Argumente für den Dualismus vom Standpunkt eines Neurophysiologen. Aus Forschung und Medizin 5(1): 9–24.

Eckert W.P. (1981). Leben und Werk des Hl. Albertus Magnus. In: A. Fries, ed., Albertus

Magnus: Ausgewählte Texte. Lateinisch-Deutsch. Darmstadt: Wissenschaftliche Buchgesellschaft, Vol. 7–30.
Eibl-Eibesfeldt I. (1970). The biology of behaviour. New York: Holt, Reinhart and Winston 530p.
Flasch K. (1986). Das philosophische Denken im Mittelalter: Von Augustin bis Machiavelli. Stuttgart: Reclam, 720p.
Fries A. (1981). Albertus Magnus: Ausgewählte Texte. Darmstadt: Wissenschaftliche Buchgesellschaft, 265p.
Gasson J.A. (1963). The internal senses: Functions or powers? The Thomist 26: 1–14.
Grabmann M. (1926/1956). Mittelalterliches Geistesleben. Abhandlungen zur Geschichte der Scholastik und Mystik. München: Beck, 3 vols.
Grüsser O.-J. (1986). Interaction of efferent and afferent signals: A history of ideas and experimental paradigms. Acta Psychologica 63: 3–21.
Grüsser O.-J. (1990). Vom Ort der Seele. In: Aus Forschung und Medizin. Streit um die Seele. Berlin: Schering, I: 75–96.
Grüsser O.-J. and Grüsser-Cornehls U. (1968). Neurophysiologische Grundlagen visueller angeborener Auslösemechanismen beim Frosch. Z vergl Physiol 59: 1–24.
Grüsser O.-J. and Hagner M. (1990). On the history of deformation phosphenes and the idea of internal light generated in the eye for the purpose of vision. Doc Ophthalmol 74: 57–85.
Grüsser O.-J. and Landis Th. (1991). Visual agnosias and other disturbances of visual perception and cognition. London: Macmillan, 610 p.
Grüsser O.-J. and Theiss P. (1992). Die Theorie des Sehens in der Naturphilosophie von Albertus Magnus. Sitzungsberichte, V. Zusammenkunft der Julius Hirschberg Gesellschaft, Dresden, 24.–27.Oktober 1991, Zbl Oph 136: 652–653.
Hagner M. (1987). Zur Geschichte vom Licht im Auge und der Physiologie des Druckphosphens im Verhältnis zu den jeweils zeitgenössischen Sehtheorien. Med. Diss., Berlin: Freie Universität, 164p.
Harvey R. (1975). The inward wits: Psychological theories in the Middle Ages and the Renaissance. London: Warburg 79p.
Haubst R. (1952). Zum Fortleben Alberts des Grossen bei Heymerich von Kamp und Nikolaus von Kues. Münster i.W.: Aschendorff (Studia Albertina: Suppl. IV).
Haubst R. (1980). Albert, wie Cusanus ihn sah. In: G. Meyer and A. Zimmermann, eds.: Albertus Magnus, Doctor Universalis. Walberberger Studien 6: 167–194.
Hering E. (1870/1912). Über das Gedächtnis als eine allgemeine Funktion der organisierten Materie. Reprint: Ostwalds Klassiker der exakten Wissenschaften, Leipzig: Reclam, Nr. 148.
Hirchberg J. (1899/1912). Geschichte der Augenheilkunde. In: Graefe-Saemisch, Handbuch der gesammten Augenheilkunde, 2nd ed. Leipzig, Vols, 12–15. Reprint, Hildesheim: Georg Olms 1977.
Janz D. (1969). Die Epilepsien: Spezielle Pathologie und Therapie. Stuttgart: Thieme.
Kepler J. (1604). Ad Vitelloni paralipomena. Reprint in: F Hammer. (ed): J. Kepler, Gesammelte Werke, München: Beck.
Kepler J. (1611). Dioptrice. In: W. Dyck and M. von Casper, eds. (1937–1963): J. Kepler, Gesammelte Werke. München: Beck.
Kopp p. (1933). Psychiatrisches bei Albertus Magnus. Z ges Neurol Psychiat 147: 50–60.
Layer A. (1980). Zeittafel zu Albert dem Grossen. In: Albert von Lauingen – 700 Jahre. Lauingen: Historischer Verein Dillingen an der Donau, pp. 21–30.
Leyhacker J. (1927). Zur Entwicklung der Lehre von den Hirnventrikeln als Sitz psychischer Vermögen. Sudhoff's Arch Gesch Med 19:253–286.
Liertz R. (1948). Albert der Grosse: Gedanken über sein Leben und aus seinen Werken. Münster i.W.: Aschendorff, 277p.
Lindberg D. (1983). Roger Bacon's philosophy of nature: A critical edition, with English translation, Introduction and notes of De multiplicatione specierum and De speculis comburentibus. Oxford: Clarendon, 420 p.
Lindberg D. (1987). Auge und Licht im Mittelalter: Die Entwicklung der Optik von Alkindi bis Kepler. Frankfurt a.M.: Suhrkamp, 573 p.

Mach E. (1885/1906). Die Analyse der Empfindungen und das Verhältnis des Physischen zum Psychischen. Jena: Fischer, 309 p. English edition; The analysis of sensations and the relation of the physical to the psychical. New York: Dover, 1959: 380 p.
McEvoy J. (1982). The philosophy of Robert Grosseteste. Oxford: Clarendon, 560 p.
Meuthen E. (1964). Nikolaus von Kues, 1401–1464: Skizze einer Biographie, 2nd ed. Münster i.W.: Aschendorff, 138p.
Ogarek P.J.S. (1931). Die Sinneserkenntnis Alberts des Grossen verglichen mit derjenigen des Thomas von Aquin. Theol. Diss. Lwów, 163p.
Ostler H. (1906). Die Psychologie des Hugo von St. Victor. Ein Beitrag zur Geschichte der Psychologie in der Frühscholastik. Münster i.W.: Aschendorff, 183p.
Plato (1969) 'Timaios'. In: Sämtliche Werke, Vol. 3 (ed. E. Loewenthal, 6th ed. Köln: Hegner, pp. 93–191.
Popper K.R. and Eccles J.C. (1977). The self and its brain. New York: Springer, 597 p.
Rahman F. (1952/1982). Avicenna's Psychology. London: Hyerion; Reprint: Westport, 127p.
Reylly G.C. (1934). The psychology of St. Albert the Great compared with that of St. Thomas. Theol. Diss. Washington, DC: Catholic University Press, 95p.
Russell B. (1945). A History of Western Philosophy. New York: Clarion, 895p.
Scheeben H.C. (1980). Albertus Magnus: Ordensmann, Bischof, Gelehrter, Mann des Volkes, 3rd ed. Köln; Rheinau, 182p.
Schipperges H. (1980). Das medizinische Denken bei Albertus Magnus. In: G. Meyer and A. Zimmermann, eds.: Albertus Magnus. Doctor Universalis. Walberberger Studien 6: 279–294.
Schlette H.R. (1961). Die Nichtigkeit der Welt: Der philosophische Horizont des Hugo von St. Victor. München: Kösel, 183p.
Schmidt-Degenhard M. (1990). Versteinertes Dasein: Zur Geschichte der Melancholie. Aus Forschung und Medizin 5(1): 45–56.
Schneider A. (1903). Die Psychologie Alberts des Grossen. Beiträge zur Geschichte der Philosophie des Mittelalters, Vols. 4–6. Münster i.W.: Aschendorff.
Siraisi N.G. (1980). The medical learning of Albertus Magnus. In: J. Weisheipl, ed.: Albertus Magnus and the Sciences. Commemorative Essays. Toronto: Pontifical Institute of Medieval Studies. pp. 379–404.
Sperling G. (1967). Successive approximations to a model of short term memory. Acta Psychologica 27: 285–292.
Steneck N.H. (1970). The problem of the internal senses in the fourteenth century. Phil. Diss. Wisconsin; University of Wisconsin, 323p.
Steneck H.H. (1974). Albert the Great on the classification and localization of the internal senses. Isis 63: 193–211.
Steneck N.H. (1980). Albert on the psychology of sense perception. In: J. Weisheipl, Ed.: Albertus Magnus and the Sciences. Commemorative Essays. Toronto; Pontifical Institute of Mediaeval Sciences, pp. 263–290.
Stratton G.M. (1917). Theophrastus and the Greek physiological psychology before Aristotle. New York: Allen and Unwin; Reprint Amsterdam: Bonset 1964, 227p.
Taylor J. (1957). The origin and early life of Hugh of St. Victor: An evaluation of the tradition. Notre Dame, Indiana : University of Notre Dame, 70p.
Taylor J. (1961). The Didascalicon of Hugh of St. Victor: A medieval guide of the arts. New York: Columbia University Press. 354p.
Telfer W. (1955). Cyril of Jerusalem and Nemesius of Emesa. Library of Christian Classics, Vol. 4. London: SCM Press.
Theiss P. (1994). Die Wahrnehmungspsychologie und Sinnesphysiologie bei Albertus Magnus: ein Modell der Sinnes- und Hirnfunktion aus der Zeit des Mittelalters: Mit einer Übersetzung aus 'De anima'. Med. Diss. Berlin: Freie Universität (in preparation).
Thorndike L. (1929). A history of magic and experimental science, Vol. 2. New York.
Verbeke G. and Moncho I.R. (1975). Némésius d'Emèse: De natura hominis. Leiden: Brill, 260 p.
Wallace W.A. (1980a). Albertus Magnus on the suppositional necessity in the natural sciences.

In: J. Weisheipl ed.: Albertus Magnus and the Sciences. Commemorative Essays. Toronto: Pontifical Institute of Mediaeval Sciences. pp. 103–128.
Wallace W.A. (1980b). The scientific methodology of St. Albert the Great. In: G. Mayer and A. Zimmermann, eds.: Albertus Magnus, Doctor Universalis. Walberberger Studien 6: 385–407.
Weiseipl J. (1980). The life and works of St. Albert the Great. In: J. Weisheipl, ed.: Albertus Magnus and the Sciences. Commemorative Essays. Toronto: Pontifical Institute of Mediaeval Studies, pp. 13–49.
Wolfson H.A. (1935). The internal senses in Latin, Arabic, and Hebrew philosophic texts. Harvard Theol Rev 28: 69–133.

Address for correspondence: Prof. Otto-Joachim Grüsser, Department of Physiology, Freie Universität, Armimallee 22, D-14195 Berlin, Germany
Phone: (30) 838 2543; Fax: (30) 838 2507

Documenta Ophthalmologica **86**: 153–161, 1994.

Further studies by Christoph Scheiner concerning the optics of the eye

F. DAXECKER
University Eye Clinic, Innsbruck, Austria

Key words: History of ophthalmology, Anatomy of the eye, Physiological optics, Rotational centre of the eye, Visual angle

Abstract. The physician, mathematician and astronomer was born in 1573 in Wald near Mindelheim in Swabia, Germany. He died in 1650 in Neisse in Silesia. He discovered the sun spots and also dealt with the physiological optics of the eye. Further observations of Scheiner's are represented, i.e. from his books *Oculus* and *Rosa Ursina*, concerning the anatomy of the eye, the crossing of the beams through a small opening (Camera obscura), stenopeic effect, proof that the crossing of the visual beams takes place in the eye, description of the cataract and its treatment, Christoph Scheiner's eye model, the visual angle, the rotational centre of the eye, the comparison of the optics of the eye and the telescope.

Introduction

The physician, mathematician and astronomer Christoph Scheiner SJ was born in Wald near Mindelheim, Swabia in 1573 and died in Neisse, Silesia in 1650. During his lifetime, the telescope was invented, implying enormous progress for science. Scheiner discovered the sun spots and was also engaged in the physiological optics of the eye. A comprehensive report on his life was given in 1992 in Documenta Ophthalmologica [1]. In that paper, the following discoveries by Scheiner regarding the physiological optics of the eye were dealt with: radius of curvature of the cornea, nasal exit of the optic nerve, increase in the radius of curvature of the lens in case of accommodation, light reaction of the pupil, narrowing of the pupil in case of accommodation, Scheiner's Procedure (double images in case of ametropia), refractive indices of the various parts of the eye, Scheiner's Experiment (proof of the reversed retinal image).

There are also further observations and developments of Scheiner's regarding the optics of the eye which are represented subsequently. These physiological and physical experiments are taken from Scheiner's book *Oculus* [2] and from his main work, *Rosa Ursina* [3]. Parts of *Oculus* are available in a German version [5], the figures taken from *Oculus* are in original size, Fig. 5 is scaled down.

Scheiner's discoveries

Description of the anatomy of the eye

The book *Oculus* is subdivided into three books of two parts each. In the first part of the book, Scheiner describes the anatomy of the eye, and he still assumes seven eye muscles [2, 4]. Apart from the description of the individual parts of the eye like cornea, lens, sclera, uvea, ciliary processes and optic nerve, he also supplies exact instructions for the section of the eye: 'The eye, however, is cut, either in raw state or somewhat filled up with warm water. Full boiling is likely to make it unsuitable for this particular purpose. If it is nevertheless immersed into boiling water, it is thus prepared to differentiate its individual shells. Since the heat dissolves the glueing binders, the parts can be considered separately' *Oculus*, p. 26).[1]

Crossing of beams through a small opening (camera obscura) [6]

Here he submits the proof of the crossing of the light beams and proves that the beams run linearly according to the laws of the light and that they cross behind the small opening and not in front of it. In this connection he writes in *Oculus*, p. 32 (Fig. 1): 'ABC be the eye in front of which the dark screen DEFG, consisting of any material, but provided with a small hole, is put; through this hole, the visual object IK, located behind the screen, shall catch the eye. This will happen through the beams IHL and KHM, which cross in the hole H. All that is proved by the following observation: if another impervious small screen NO or something similar be gradually shifted towards the opening H between the eye and the screen mentioned, it can be perceived that point I of the visual object will disappear before the

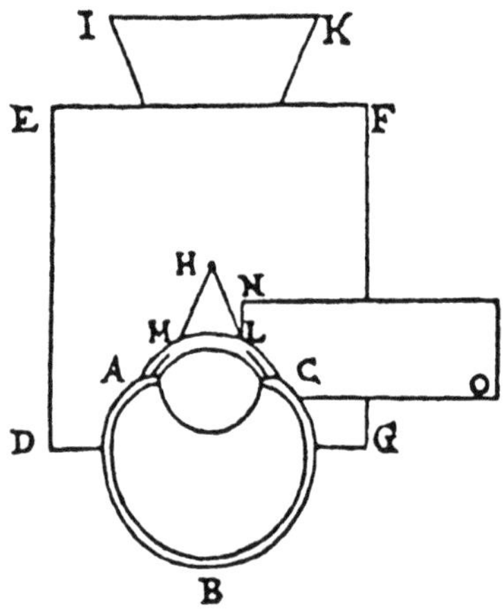

Fig. 1. Crossing of beams in a small hole-camera obscura. Explanation in the text.

small screen itself has reached the hole as such' [6]. He further states: '.... 'Should the small screen not be moved to the hole between the eye and the screen EFGD, but behind the latter, the relation with regard to the position will not reverse when obscured and the obscured object and the obscured small screen will be on the same side of the eye and the object. From this results that the beams IL and KM do not cross on the other side, but on this side of the opening H, namely between the eye and the screen EG' (*Oculus*, p. 33).[2]

Stenopeic effect

Christoph Scheiner also observed the corrective effect of the stenopeic hole, which makes the image appear more clearly and smaller to the myopic person: 'The object seen through the hole appears somewhat smaller than when seen without the aid of the hole, but it is perceived in a far more exact, sharp, and determined way' (*Oculus* p. 34).[3]

Proof that the crossing of the visual beams takes place in the eye
Christoph Scheiner describes a man, whose lens of the left eye was turbid and, in addition, temporally subluxated. Through the gap remaining free nasally, the patient was able to see and Scheiner was able to prove that temporally located objects could be perceived. He proves this by means of a figure (Fig. 2). This figure as well as the corresponding description are to be found on page 36 of his book *Oculus*. He writes in this connection: 'Here ABC is the iris of the eye, DEFG the pupil, DHFG the white small cloud obscuring the pupil, DEFH the permeable sickle. Already when the eye looks upon opposite objects, it perceives these in reverse and changed application. Thus, for example, if ILNK is assumed as the object, it is not point I which is perceived through the sickle, but point K by means of the beam HK which is completely oblique to the sickle'.[4]

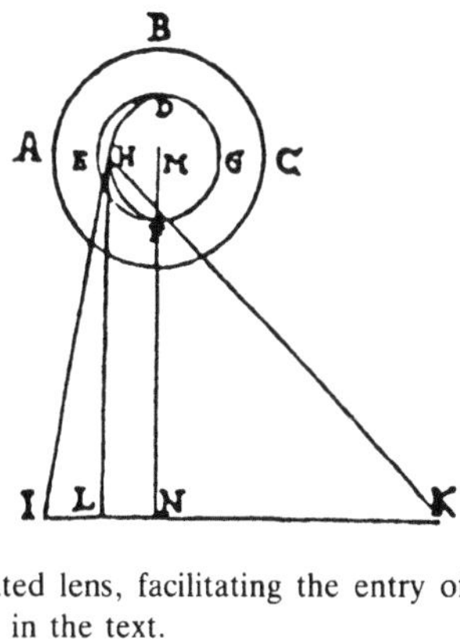

Fig. 2. An eye with a subluxated lens, facilitating the entry of light into the eye through a sickle-shaped gap. Explanation in the text.

Description of the cataract and its treatment

Scheiner does here reflect the opinion on the formation of the cataract, common in his time, as well as the usual operative therapy, where the lens is luxated into the vitreous body (per depressionem) [7]. In this connection Christoph Scheiner writes: 'There are people who are deprived of their vision by a thin skin, laying itself in front of the pupil originating from the fluid of the eye between the cornea and the crystal lens. This results in the fact that the shapes of the visual objects, are prevented from entering into the eye, so that the eye is deprived of any ability of perceiving them. Therefore the surgeons, called upon for help, apply the following treatment against this evil. With a silver needle they penetrate the cornea laterally, tear that damaging thin skin down from above, wind it around the needle and immerse it into the deeper ground of the fluid of the eye in order to thus open the hole in the uvea again and permit the free passage through the pupil. If this has been achieved, the needle is pulled out and the eye is cured and apt for vision as previously,' (*Oculus*, p. 47).[5]

Eye model

Scheiner also created an eye model, consisting of a vitreous cornea, pure water as fluid of the eye, a vitreous or natural lens, and a vitreous, spherical retina. According to his description, the vitreous body is filled with air, however. He describes this eye model (Fig. 3) as follows: 'F be a burning candle, ABC a hollow glass, bordered by spherical surfaces, LMN a complete vitreous or crystalline lens; in a similar way, ASC be the surface of a glass flash and these parts be connected with each other and arranged in such a way as the parts of the eye. The front sinus be filled up with common water, the rear sinus MS with pure and clear air, however. The candle F be located in a distance of less than the length of a finger and it will shine through two openings D and E; if you hold a clean sheet of paper against the bordering wall OPRS then, you will catch two very clear shapes of the one flame F, namely that on the right-hand side through the right opening D and that on the left-hand-side through the left opening E' (*Oculus*, p. 66).[6]

The visual angle (*Angulus visorius*, *visual field*)

Christoph Scheiner makes the beams, originating from the end points of an object, cross at the rear pole of the lens and calls the angle so developing the visual angle. These beams do then hit the retina and he believes (erroneously) that in the retina (of finite thickness) that part of the beam which penetrates the retina permits the determination of the direction from which the object is seen [8, 9]. He writes: 'When the object AB is perceived, its visible basis will be on the retina CD. Basically the irradiated part is so big that it corresponds to the distance AB from the visual object. The visual

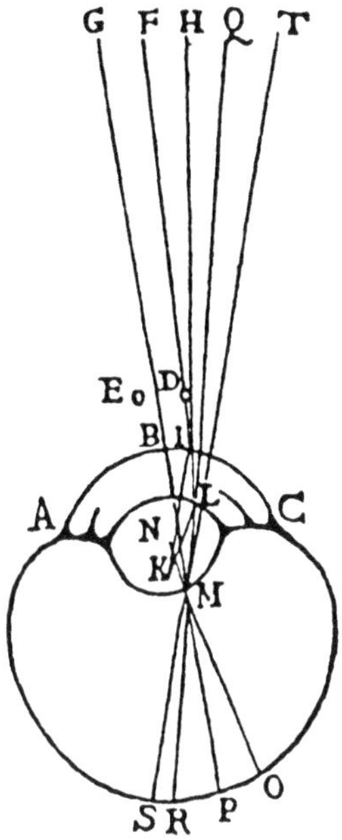

Fig. 3. Christoph Scheiner's Eye Model. The explanation is given in the text.

beams proper may be DE and CF, parts of the beams HD and IC; therefore the visual angle does exist in the eye' (*Oculus*, p. 221, Fig. 4.)[7]

Rotational centre of the eye

Christoph Scheiner recognized quite correctly that the eye can move like a sphere inside a surrounding capsule. This recognition fell into oblivion and was rediscovered again 200 years later [8–10]. Christoph Scheiner writes: 'Thus the eye revolves spherically in its socket around its own centre which

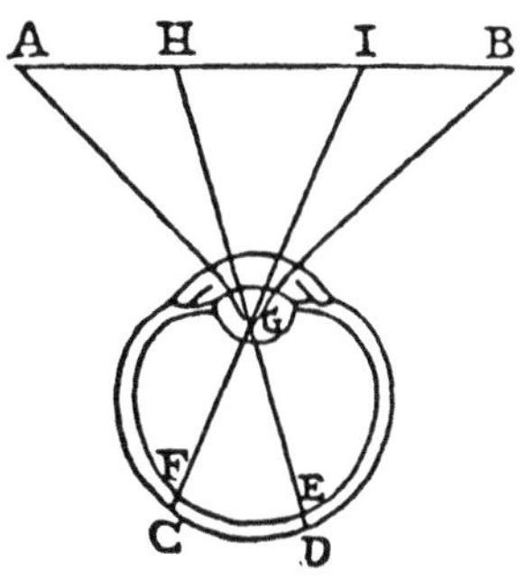

Fig. 4. The light beams originate from the end points of an object, cross at the rear pole of the lens and hit the retina.

coincides with the centre of the vitreous body, the border membrane, the choroid, the retina and finally the sclera' (*Oculus*, p. 245).[8]

Comparison of the optics of the eye and the telescope in 'Rosa Ursina Sive Sol'

The book *Rosa Ursina Sive Sol* appeared in Rome between 1626 and 1630. It is subdivided into four sections. The second section (Liber secundus) is subdivided into 42 chapters. First Scheiner deals with the helioscope for the observation of the sun. From chapter 23 onwards he compares the eye with a telescope and presents in that connection a beautiful copperplate engraving (Fig. 5). This part of the book extends from page 106 to 123 and can therefore be quoted in a few basic points only. As far as Fig. 5 is concerned

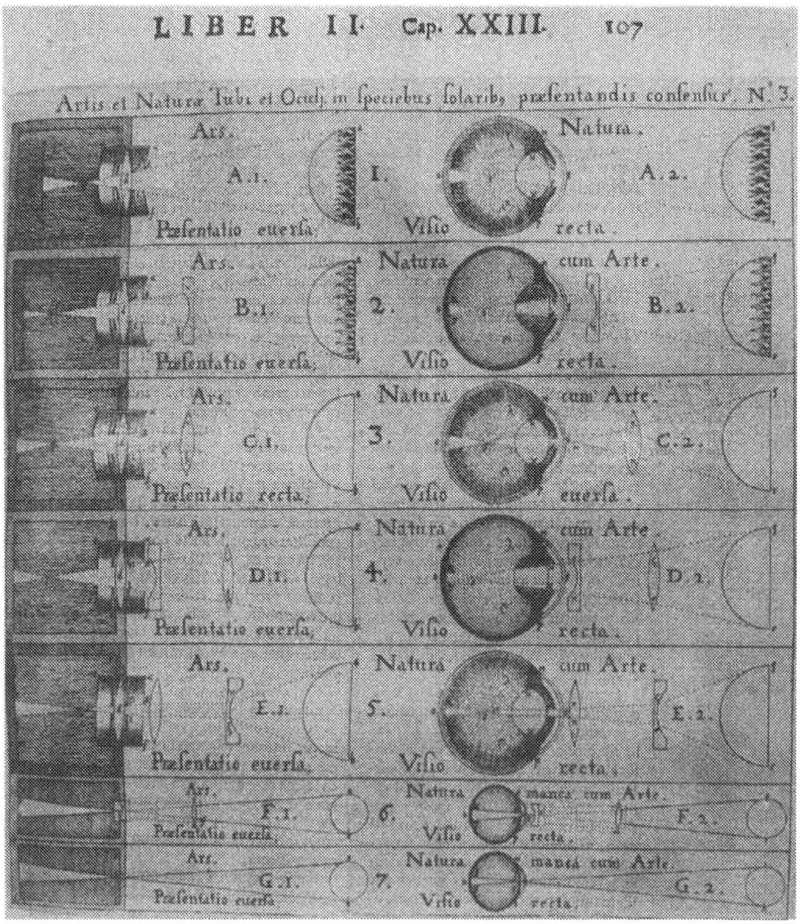

Fig. 5. The copperplate engraving is subdivided into 7 sections. On the right-hand side, optical conditions on the eye are represented respectively. The explantation is given in the text.

it is striking that he locates the crossing point of the light beams approximately in the centre of the bulbus and not, as already published in *Oculus* in 1619, at the rear pole of the lens of the eye (see Fig. 4). Furthermore it also strikes one's attention that with respect to the individual text illustrations in Fig. 5, the pupils are represented in different widths. Fig. 5 is subdivided into 7 sections (A – G):

Chapter 23 (A1, A2): Comparison of the eye with a lens; the eye as such is a system of lenses, similar to a telescope.

Chapter 24 (B1, B2): Eye and concave lens for myopic persons. The bigger the distance of the concave lens, the smaller the image; the stronger the lens, the wider the image.

Chapter 25 (C1, C2): Eye and convex lens for myopic persons. The eye is a system of two convex lenses. A convex lens can also be applied with myopic persons (does, however, develop a reverse image).

Chapter 26 (not represented in Fig. 5): Explanation of different lens combinations as a sequence of points of confusion and clearness of the image. The eye behaves like a lens. On the retina, the only visual instrument, the image develops clearly and reversely.

Chapter 27 (D1, D2): Here he discusses projection through a lens onto a screen. The retina of the eye can always be compared with the screen.

Chapter 28 (D1, D2): Concave lenses in different combinations with convex ones. A convex lens and behind it a concave one reflects the image bigger than a convex one alone. Application when making observations of the sun. He describes the Dutch telescope.

Chapter 29 (D1, D2): The Dutch telescope. Convex and concave lenses. Myopic persons alter the distance between the lenses. Because of the smallness of the pupil, the eye cannot take up the entire image. As far as Fig. 5 is concerned, he does not describe E1 and E2 in the text. This figure represents the reverse Dutch telescope which leads to a diminution of the image. Likewise he does not describe F2 showing the arrangement of the Dutch telescope with an aphakic eye.

Chapter 30 (G1, G2): G1 shows the representation of the camera obscura with reversed image and G2 the representation of the aphakic eye with upright image.

In chapters 31 and 32 he deals with his observations of the sun and the moon.

In chapters 33 he supplies instructions for the assembly of a telescope: a plane-convex objective is to be given preference likewise as a plane-convex ocular.

In chapters 34 to 42 he describes the technique of sun observation.

Notes

1. Secatur autem oculus vel crudus, vel aqua calida nonnihil constipatus. Nam licet elixatio plena ipsum huic rei inutilem reddat, mersus tamen in feruentem, tunicis discernendis adaptatur. Quia calor glutinosa vincula resoluit, partesq; dissimiles in conspectum dat, &c.

2. Sit oculus ABC, cui obtendatur lamina opaca DEFG, è quacunque materia exili foramine H pertusa, quo res visilis IK trans laminam sita, in ipsum veniat; fiet id per radios IHL, & KHM, decussatos ad foramen H, quod probatur hac experientia. Si intra oculum & laminam dictam, alia lamella NO opaca vel aliud quid simile sensim admoueatur versus foramé H, animaduertetur rei visilis punctum I occultari, antequam lamella ipsum foramen ex illa parte attigerit. ... Si lamella non inter oculum & laminam, EFGD, sed post ipsam foramini adhibeatur; non permutabitur in occultando situs, sed res occultata; & lamella occultas erunt ad eandem partem oculi & obiecti, ex quo patet, ràdios IL & KM. no trans, sed cis foramen H decussari, inter oculum videlicet & laminam EG.
3. Res per foramen aspecta, minor quidem apparet, quam absque foraminis adminiculo, multo tamen praecisior, distinctior, & accuratior apprehenditur.
4. In qua Iris oculi est ABC, pupilla DEFG, nubecula alba pupillae obducta DHFG, falx perspicua DEFH. Iam si oculus iste rest obiectas intuetur, in oppositis & permutatis stibus eas conspicatur; vt in exemplo, si obiectum statuatur ILNK, punctum I non videbitur a lunula DEFH, sed punctum K per radium HK.
5. Svnt homines aliqui, quibus obtutum aufert, tenuis quaedeam pellicula, e viscolo humoreintra tunicam Corneam & humorem Crystallinum pupillae obducta: quae facit vt rerum aspectabilium formae ingressu oculi exclusae, eundem facultate illas percipiendi omni destituant: vnde Chirurgi in auxilium aduocati huic malo hanc medicinam faciunt. Acu argentea tunicam Corneam ex latere perfodiunt, tunicellamque illam adulterinam supernè detractam circa acum conuoluunt, & in inferiores humoris aquei sinus mergunt, vt hac ratione foramine Vueae denuo patefacto, liber transitus in pupillam detur. quo obtento, extrahitur acus & oculus curatus est, atque rebus videndis, vt ante idoneus.
6. F, sit candela ardens, ABC vitru sphaericum cauu, LMN, lens vel vitrea, vel Crystallina solida; ASC, esto similiter superficies ampullae vitrea, & sind haecita coniuncta, atque disposita uti partes oculi, & sinum anteriorem LB impleat aqua naturalis, posteriorem MS purus putusque aer, adhibeatur candela F interuallo IF minore quam sit longitudo digiti, traluceatque per duo foramina D & E, quo facto, si in fundo OPRS chartam mundam obieceris, excipies vnius faculae F duas distinctissimas formas, & dextramquidem per dextrum foramen D, sinistram per sinistru E.
7. Vt si obiectum AB videatur, erit basis visoria in Retina CD; tanta videlicet in eius fundo depicta portio, quanta proportionaliter basi AB rei visibilis respondet. & radij formaliter visorii erunt segmenta DE atque CF radiotum HD, atque IC; beneficio igitur portionum DE atq; CF, angulus visorius in oculo existit.
8. Sic motus oculi in suo foramine positi est sphaericus, super suimet centrum, quod idem est cum centro humoris Vitrei, tunicae Hyaloydis, Choroidis, Retinae, ac demum Sclerodis posticae.

References

1. Daxecker, F. (1992). Christoph Scheiner's eye studies. Documenta Ophthalmologica 81: 27–35.
2. Scheiner Ch. (1619). Oculus hoc est: Fundamentum opticum. Oeniponti. Apud Danielem Agricolam.
3. Scheiner Ch. (1626–1630). Rosa Ursina Sive Sol. Braccioni, Apud Andream Phaecum Typographum Ducalem.
4. Ziggelaar A., SJ (1983). François de Aguilón SJ (1567–1617) Scientist and Architect. Bibliotheca Instituti Historici S.J. (Rome), Vol. 44, p. 105.
5. von Rohr, M. (1919). Ausgewählte Stücke aus Christoph Scheiners Augenbuch, Zeitschrift für ophthalmologische Optik 7:35–44, 53–64, 76–91, 101–113; 121–133.
6. Goercke, E. (1992). Christoph Scheiners Versuche mit der 'Camera obscura', In: Die Jesuiten in Ingolstadt, p. 144, (1549–1773), Stadtarchiv Ingolstadt.

7. Hirschberg, J. (1908). Geschichte der Augenheilkunde. In: Graefe Saemisch Handbuch der gesamten Augenheilkunde, Vol. 13, Leipzig: W. Engelmann, pp. 284, 373.
8. Mauthner, L. (1876). Vorlesungen über die optischen Fehler des Auges. Wien: W. Braumüller, pp. 121–122.
9. Daxecker, F. (1993). Der Naturwissenschaftler Christoph Scheiner SJ in der optischen Literatur. Ein medizinhistorischer Beitrag. Ber. nat.-med. Verein Innsbruck, Vol. 80 (in press).
10. von Rohr, M. (1915). Das Auftreten des Augendrehpunktes in der Physiologie und in der technischen Optik. Zeitschrift für Instrumentenkunde 35(8): 187–215.

Address for correspondence: Univ. Prof. Dr. Franz Daxecker, University Eye Clinic, Anichstraße 35, A-6020 Innsbruck, Austria
Phone: (512) 504 3731; Fax: (512) 504 3722

Documenta Ophthalmologica **86**: 163–166, 1994.

On the invention of the ophthalmoscope

ROBERT WEALE
Moorfields Eye Hospital, and Age Concern Institute of Gerontology, King's College, London, UK

Key words: History of ophthalmology, Ophthalmoscopy, Optics, Purkinje, Visual science

Abstract. The author offers an English translation of three passages of Purkinje's *Commentatio de examine physiologico organi visus* (1823). He shows that Purkinje made three inventions: (1) by using a transparent mirror, (2) by anticipating Maxwellian illumination, and (3) by providing the first recorded ophthalmic examination of animal and human eyes.

In his centennial appreciation of Sir William Bowman, Patrick Trevor-Roper [1] referred to his early use of the ophthalmoscope. In attributing the invention of the instrument to Charles Babbage, Trevor-Roper followed the tradition stamped on our ideas by Duke-Elder [2]. Either Duke-Elder quoted without having consulted the original (which would not have been a unique occurrence), or else he failed to seek the help of someone whose Latin was better than his own. Otherwise he could not have missed the passage following the one in which Purkinje carefully describes how he obtained his eponymous images.

Some time ago I leafed idly through a facsimile copy of Purkinje's writings [3], in which he described the use of these images, which are illustrated there by amazing engravings. After the description of how he obtained them there appears the following passage:

> Limpiditas vel turbatio corporis vitrei externe ex nigredine pupillae aut integra aut nebulosa cognoscitur, distinctis obliqua inspectione et illuminatione juxta methodos prius adnotatas, quae humori aqueo aut lenti pertinent.
>
> Ast cavum quoque oculi ubi corpus vitreum residet justa methodo inspicere casu mihi datum est, dum perspiciliis myopum armatus, canis oculum, candelae lumine a tergo ejus e longinquo lucente, eo scopo inquisivissem, ut de natura splendoris, qui non raro ex canum feliumque oculis miro modo promanat, edocerer. En! quoties certa directione oculum caniculi inspexissem, lumen illud percellens apparebat, donec fontem invenirem lumen e cavitate vitri in interna oculi reflexum indeque iterum retroflexum. Eodem statim in hominibus experimento repetito idem phaenomenon oblatum est, pupilla namque integra laeto aurantio colore lucebat. De sedo adhuc luminis reflexi in dubio versans oculum

artificialem conficiendum curavi, cujus cavum aqua limpida aut diversis gradibus turbida repletum posteriorem parientem, simulque liquidi substantiam reflexo lumine referebat.

Iam itaque nulla fere oculi membrana aut substantia interna liquidi, lumine rite reflexo oculoque inspicienti latebit, quae si practici anxiam fere physiologorum inquisitionem spernentes non despicient aut perhorrescent non sine usu in oculum Diagnostica invenient.

The dying embers of a flickering Latin might render this as follows:

'The clarity or turbidity of the vitreous body [ocular interior] can be noted from the outside by the blackness or haziness of the entire pupil, and, by the different methods described earlier, oblique illumination and inspection can determine whether the conditions reside in the aqueous humour or the lens.

'Moreover, I chanced to examine by the appropriate method also the region of the eye occupied by the vitreous body; furnished with glasses worn by myopes, I inspected the eye of a dog in order to discover the cause of the brilliance spreading frequently from the eyes of dogs and cats. The illumination was provided by a candle shining from afar behind the animal. Lo and behold! when I examined the puppy's eye from a given direction, a very bright light kept appearing, till I found as its source light deflected into the eye and, in turn, reflected from the vitreous chamber. Having at once determined to repeat the experiment on man, the same phenomenon appeared, that is to say the entire pupil glowed with a golden colour. Still in doubt about the precise location of the source of this reflexion, I though it advisable to construct an artificial eye: with clear water or varying degrees of turbidity filling the cavity and reaching its posterior wall, the reflected light reappeared at once through the substance of the liquid.

'Henceforth hardly any ocular tissue or internal substance of the fluid will remain concealed from the examining eye when properly illuminated; and, if practitioners were not to reject, look down on, and shudder at, the anxious

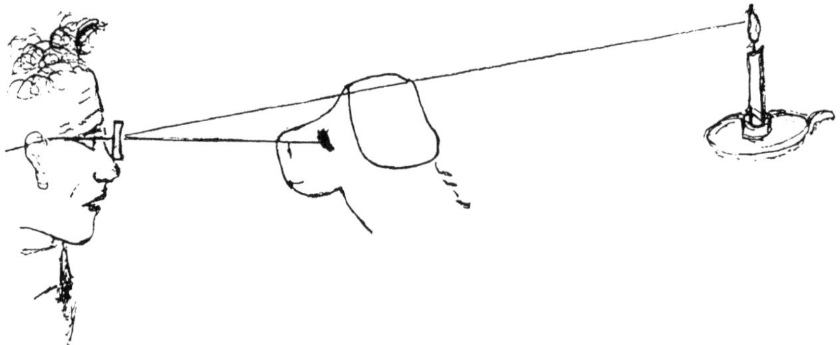

Fig. 1. Scheme of Purkinje's arrangement for examining the ocular interior as deduced from his descript

inquiries of physiologists they might not find them without use in ocular diagnoses.'

Figure 1 is my illustration of what I think Purkinje is stating in the second paragraph in the above passage.

The final crack is a Purkinje perennial: on the occasion of the delivery of his inaugural lecture as professor of physiology at the University of Prague he concluded by saying that a knowledge of physiology would make doctors poorer but better.

But what about the substance of the translated passage? It contains three

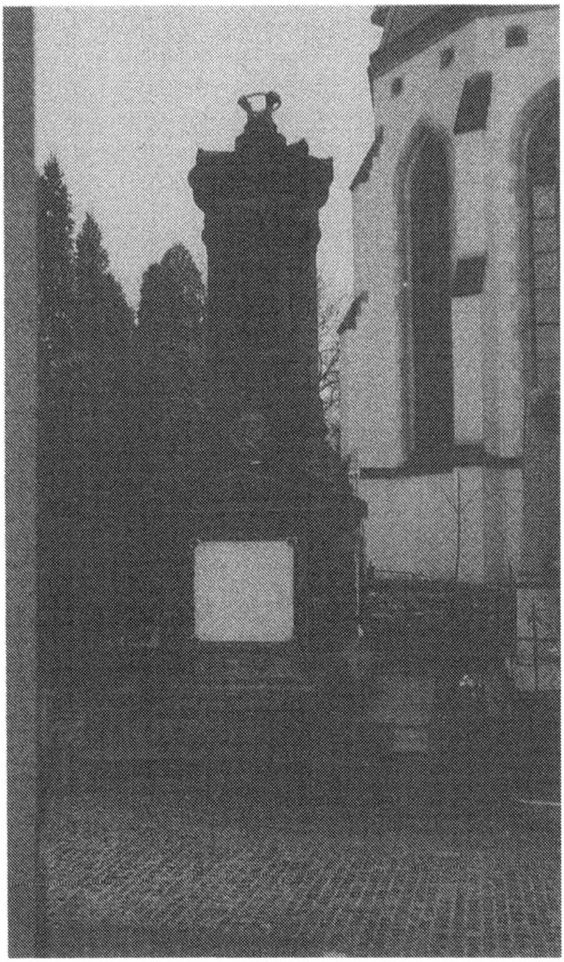

Fig. 2. The tomb of Jan Purkinje (note the unteutonized spelling of his name).

inventions two of which were not essential to the successful operation of Purkinje's experimental arrangement for viewing the ocular interior. Purkinje made use of a transparent mirror, which does not appear to have been described any earlier. Helmholtz [4] used it later, but did not acknowledge Purkinje's priority.

Purkinje anticipated Maxwellian illumination, the principle of which involves imaging a light source in the plane of the entrance pupil of an optical device, which is the most economic method of illuminating a surface behind such a pupil. If that were not so, the use of a distant candle coupled with a myopic correction which would have had a concave reflecting surface would be hard to understand. Finally, Purkinje had grasped the notion that, for an eye to be examined, entrance and exit beams have to be virtually collinear. He combined these elements in the first recorded ophthalmoscopic examination of animal and human eyes. It may be noted that the significance of the first two of these innovations escaped Julius Hirschberg [5]. who, as I have been advised since the acceptance of this paper for publication, had prepared a German translation of the Latin text. Since this does not seem to have reached the Anglo-Saxon consciousness, [1] there can be little harm in offering one in English.

Like his countryman, Mendel, Purkinje has not been in the forefront of receiving credit for his work. He rests in a famous Prague burial-ground, a mixture of London's Highgate Cemetery and Westminster Abbey. Could it be that a perceptive designer of tombs shaped Purkinje's in the form of a handle of an ophthalmoscope (Fig. 2)?

References

1. Trevor-Roper, P. (1992). Sir William Bowman, British Journal of Ophthalmology 76: 129.
2. Duke-Elder, Sir W.S. (1962). System of ophthalmology, Vol. 7, p. 290. The foundations of ophthalmology. London: Henry Kimpton.
3. Purkinje, J.E. (1823). Commentatio de examine physiologico organi visus [Vratislaviae 1823]. The Hague: Dr W. Junk Publishers, Reprinted 1937.
4. Helmholtz, H. von (1851). Beschreibung eines Augenspiegels zur Untersuchung der Netzhaut im lebenden Auge. Berlin.
5. Hirschberg, J. (1918). Handbuch der gesammten Augenheilkunde, Vol. 15, pp. 92–95. Berlin: J. Springer.

Address for correspondence: Dr Robert Weale, Moorefield Eye Hospital, City Road, London EC1 2PJ, UK
Phone: (71) 253 3411; Fax: (71) 872 3235

Documenta Ophthalmologica **86**: 167–171, 1994.

D.B. Kagenaar and the ophthalmometer by Javal-Schiøtz

I. DEN TONKELAAR, G.K. VAN LEERSUM & H.E. HENKES
F.C. Donders Institute of Ophthalmology Utrecht, The Netherlands

Key words: History of Ophthalmology, Ophthalmometer, Instrumentmaker

Abstract: In the years 1881–1890 the Utrecht instrumentmaker D.B. Kagenaar, laboratory attendant of Donders and Snellen, played an important role in the introduction on the German market of the ophthalmometer developed by Javal and Schiøtz.

In 1864 F.C. Donders described astigmatism as a common disorder of vision that can be corrected by means of cylindrical lenses [1]. Since that time, there was a need to measure astigmatism quickly and accurately.

Ten years earlier, in 1853, H. von Helmholtz developed an ophthalmometer aimed at the exact measurement of the curvatures of the cornea and the lens [2]. By means of this instrument Helmholtz, shortly after A. Cramer [3], discovered that the curvature of the lens increases at accommodation. This instrument was perfectly suitable for scientific research, but it did not fulfil the needs of the ophthalmologist interested in routine measurement of the corneal curvature.

In 1872 E.A. Coccius developed a modification of Helmholtz' ophthalmometer intended for the ophthalmic praxis [4]. Coccius' instrument, however, remained unknown, probably because he did not attend international congresses to demonstrate his instrument. Moreover, his publication [4] was difficult to understand and the instrument seems to have missed fine workmanship [5].

Almost 10 years later, E. Javal from Paris and H. Schiøtz from Norway introduced an instrument, which they also called 'ophthalmometer', to measure astigmatism quickly, simply and accurately [6]. Although their instrument was constructed on the principles laid down by Coccius, Javal only casually refers to him. Schiøtz, on the other hand, in 1881 gave Coccius the credits he merited [5]. The first model by Javal was introduced in 1880 [7] and the second model, which he developed together with Schiøtz, was presented at the ophthalmological congresses in London and Paris in 1881 [6]. The instrument was made by the Paris instrumentmaker Laurent. The ophthalmometer by Javal and Schiøtz soon found acceptance in many European countries and the USA. In Germany, however, the instrument was very rarely used. According to Nuel and Leplat, two French colleagues of Javal, the reason for this was that the German ophthalmologists associated the name 'ophthalmometer' with their well-known, but unpractical Helmholtz ophthalmometer. In addition the term for delivery of the French instrument was often one or two years and the price was quite high: 350 French francs or 300 German Marks [8].

The Utrecht instrumentmaker D.B. Kagenaar (1842–1924) (Fig. 1), laboratory attendant of Donders and Snellen, however, succeeded to enter the German market with a modification of Javal's instrument (Fig. 2). Javal used a double-refracting quartz prism in order to produce the double images. Kagenaar replaced the quartz prism by a double prism of glass, because the quartz prism was not always available in sufficient size and purity [9]. Javal criticized the use of the double prism of glass. According to him this prism caused problems when the ophthalmometer was used by an astigmatic investigator (which he was). He also criticized Kagenaar's scale giving the direction of astigmatism which indicates 0° for the vertical and −90° and +90° for the left and right horizontal respectively, instead of 90° for the vertical and 0° and 180° for the left and right horizontal respectively [10]. However, despite his criticism, Javal mentions that Kagenaar played an important role in the distribution of the instrument on the German market

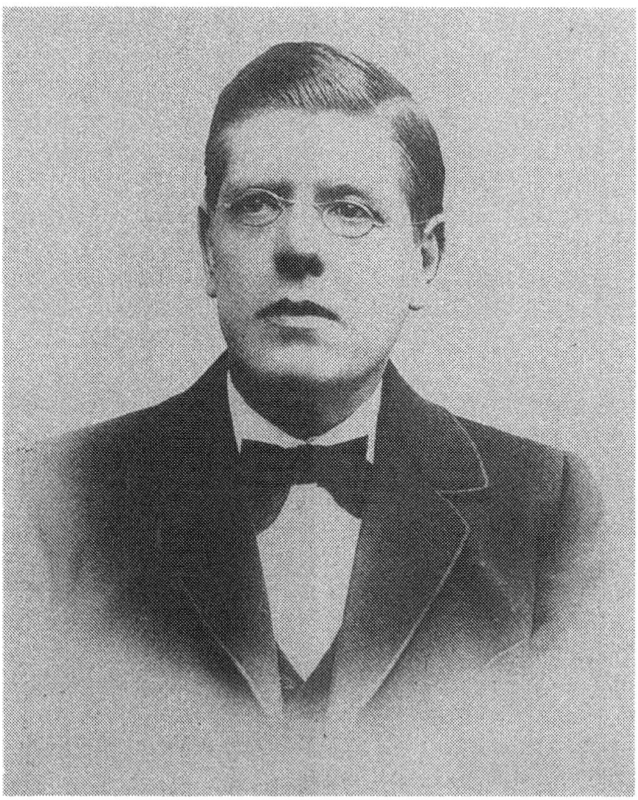

Fig. 1. D.B. Kagenaar (1842–1924).

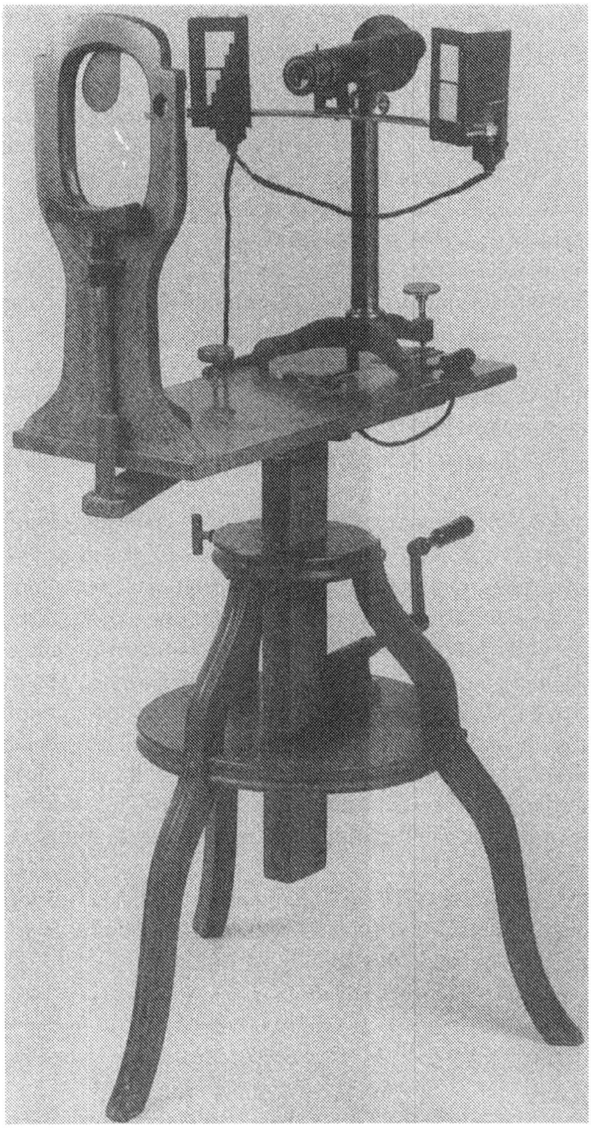

Fig. 2. An electrified astigmometer of Kagenaar of the late 19th century.

[11]. Kagenaar was Donders' instrumentmaker for over thirty years. He had his catalogues published in German and named the instrument 'astigmometer'. In the Netherlands the instrument was so well-known that it was called "the Kagenaar". Kagenaar probably was the main manufacturer of ophthalmometers (i.e. astigmometers) for the German market between 1881 and 1890. Until 1890 the only other manufacturers of ophthalmometers were

those in Paris, namely Laurent, Giroux and Goubeaux, and some manufacturers in the USA [10].

In a publication of 1901 Javal erroneously mentions that Kagenaar had delivered not more than 200 astigmometers in total [10]. Kagenaar, however, published lists of his customers in his catalogues. From those lists it appears that in 1900 Kagenaar had delivered 414 astigmometers, of which 155 were sent to Germany. He delivered not only to ophthalmologists but also to well-known dealers in various countries.

Concerning the British market a report in the ophthalmic review of 1891 reveals that the ophthalmometer by Javal-Schiøtz was hardly used in the United Kingdom [12]. In his 'mémoires d'ophtalmométrie' in 1890 Javal gives a review of the success of his instrument in various countries: the USA, Switzerland, Germany, Italy and the Scandinavian countries, but he doesn't even mention the United Kingdom [11]. In Kagenaar's catalogue of 1900, however, 37 deliveries of ophthalmometers to the United Kingdom are listed.

Between 1881 and 1911 Kagenaar delivered about 660 astigmometers [13]. Apparently Kagenaar was able to combine an average production of 22 ophthalmometers a year (and many other instruments!) with his appointment as a laboratory attendant and instrumentmaker at the laboratory of physiology of the university of Utrecht. His appointment at the university was obviously no hindrance to him for commercial success. He even took advantage of his situation by advertising that he was an instrumentmaker of the university and that he was also the laboratory attendant of such famous Utrecht professors as Donders, Snellen, Engelmann, Pekelharing, Zwaardemaker, etcetera. He also advertised that prof. dr. H. Snellen was prepared to check the ophthalmometer if so desired (presumably in order to convince hesitant buyers) [13].

In conclusion in the years 1881–1890 Kagenaar played an important role in the introduction on the German market of the ophthalmometer developed by Javal and Schiøtz.

References

1. Donders F.C. (1864). On the anomalies of accommodation and refraction of the eye. London: The New Sydenham Society, pp. 455, 501.
2. Helmholtz H. (1853). Monatsberichte der Berliner Akademie, Februar 1853, p. 137.
3. Tonkelaar den I., Henkes H.E., Leersum van G.K. (1990). Antonie Cramer's explanation of accommodation. Doc Ophthalmol 74: 87–93.
4. Coccius E.A. (1872). Ophthalmometrie und Spannungsmessung am kranken Auge. Leipzig.
5. Hirschberg J. (1918). Geschichte der Augenheilkunde, §1035, p. 166.
6. Javal E., Schiotz H. (1881). Un ophtalmomètre pratique. Annales d'Oculistique 86: 5–15.
7. Javal E. (1880). Berichte der 7. Versammlung DOG, p. 25.
8. Nuel, Leplat (1889). Astigmatisme et ophtalmométrie. Annales d'Oculistique 101: 164.

9. Van der Spil (1889). Bepaling van astigmatisme met den ophthalmometer van Javal-Schiøtz, Utrecht, p. 5
10. Javal E. (1901). Die Prüfung des Ophthalmometers. Albr. v. Graefe's Archiv f. Ophthalmologie, Bd. 52, Abt. 3, p. 539.
11. Javal E. (1890). Mémoires d'ophtalmométrie, Paris, p. VI.
12. Story B. (1891). L'ophtalmomètre dans la pratique. Annales d'Oculistique, Tome 106.
13. Kagenaar D.B. (1911). Astigmometer nach Javal und Schiøtz. Catalogue.

Address for correspondence: I. den Tonkelaar, F.C. Donders Institute of Ophthalmology. P.O. Box 85.500, 3508 GA Utrecht, The Netherlands

Documenta Ophthalmologica **86**: 173–189, 1994.

A contribution to the history of spectacles in Croatia

VJEKOSLAV DORN
University Eye Clinic, Zagreb, Croatia

Key words: History of ophthalmology, Croatia, Spectacles

Abstract: The earliest data on spectacles in Croatia originate from the 14th century. Inventories of personal belongings and valuables of distinguished individuals testify about the existence of spectacles from the 14th century onward. Pictorial representations of spectacles and spectacle cases are found in Croatia in various forms: as a watermark in a 14th century paper, on a silver altar-piece from 1477, on paintings, frescoes and wood-cuts from the 15th century onward. A pair of 16th century spectacles are kept in Split (Poljud) and a selection of 18th to 20th century spectacles are on display in various museums in Croatia. In 17th century literature the effect of lenses on ametropia is discussed and Latin and Croatian terms for spectacles and opticians are mentioned.

The earliest data on spectacles in Croatia originate from the 14th century. The first record is found in the notary files Magnificae communitatis Jadrae, No 120. Inventarii, Busta Ia., which are kept in the Historical Archives in Zadar. On 6 February 1388, public notary Articutius de Rivignano, in the presence of distinguished witnesses, wrote the inventory 'olim venerabilis domini presbyteri Philipi de Sloradis quindam plebani ecclesiae Sancti Petri novi de platea magna Jadrae'.

In the second line on the page six of the original, marked as file 68, it is written 'item unum par oculorum de vitro' (one pair of spectacles) [1] (Fig. 1).

The first artistic representation of spectacles in Croatia is a watermark in the paper of a manuscript from St Mary's monastery in Zadar (Fig. 2). In a study of watermarks in documents and manuscripts which belong to this monastery, and under number 26 two watermarks are described [2]. One is a circle divided into four equal segments by a vertical and a horizontal line. The vertical line extends beyond the circle and forms a three-leaf cluster. The countermark is a pair of spectacles, called by German authors 'Zangenbrille'. They were named so because they resemble small pincers or sugar tongs. These spectacles belong to the group of wire spectacles which were in use from the 14th to the 16th century [3].

The watermark with the spectacles from Zadar is identical to the one found in Bourges dating from 1387 [4]. Analysis of the watermarks suggests that the manuscript originates from the mid fourteenth century, and that the figures were impressed in paper of Italian provenance [5].

In the Historical Archives in Dubrovnik, in the file 'Lamenta de intus', a claim made by Vitko Zuimović on 1 July 1450, is recorded. He claims a theft

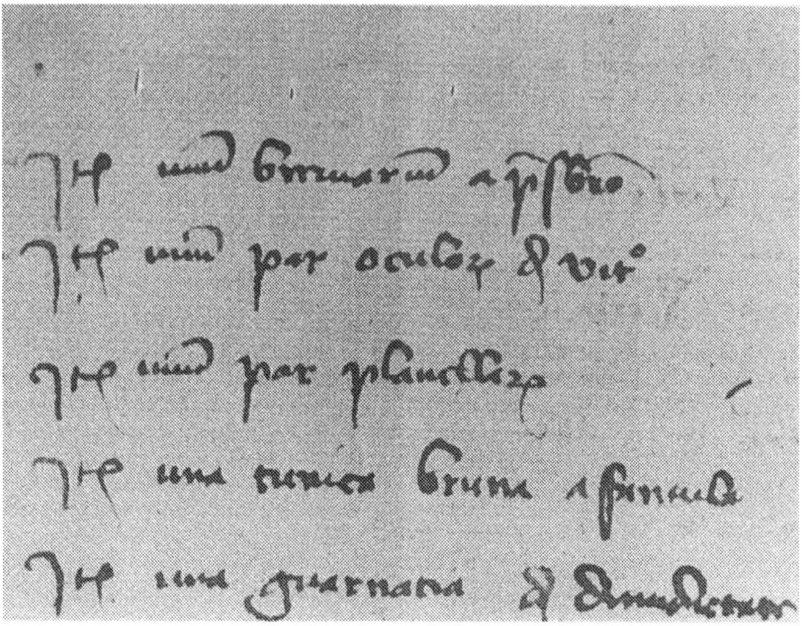

Fig. 1. The earliest Croatian record of spectacles, notary files from 1388, detail of the original (Historical Archive, Zadar).

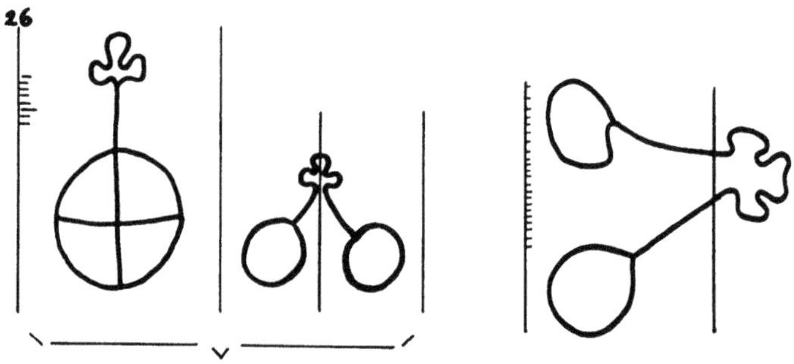

Fig. 2. Spectacles as a watermark, 14th century (St. Mary's monastery Zadar). On the right, compared with the finding from Bourges (1387), Briquet No 10621, 30 × 44.

of a silver spectacle case with a pair of spectacles, altogether 5 perpers* and 7 groschem (formerly current money) worth (... 'subtracta una capseta de argento ab ochialibus et cum ochialibus precii iperperorum quinqne...') [6].

In another document dated 24 May 1453, kept in the Historical Archives

* Perpers are silver coins in use since the 12th century in the Middle and Near East as well as on both sides of the Adriatic. In the 15th century 1 Venetian ducat = 3 perpers; 1 perper = 12 groschen.

in Dubrovnik, a silver spectacle case is mentioned ('una casella da ochiali de argento...' [7].

Beside medicine and drugs, medieval herbalists sold spectacles. This is proved by a list of objects which were to be put for auction on 13 November 1482, by Stanula, the widow of late Rikard Božidarević, aromatarius (herbalist) from Dubrovnik. Among the things to be sold were '38 pairs of fine spectacles 1 ducat and 18 groschen worth' [8].

Only very few spectacles of the oldest type have been preserved in the world. Until 1953, the shape, size and manner of use of the earliest spectacles were known only from various works of art. That year, several specimens were found in the monastery of Wienhausen near Celle in northern Germany [9].

These earliest spectacles consisted of two lenses fitted into wide wire rings (the metals used were iron, copper or brass) with a handle on one side. The ends of the handles were riveted, so that the handles formed a certain angle depending on the width of the nose. These were the so-called rivet spectacles (Nietbrille, basicles clouants) [10]. They were rather heavy and had to be held by hand as they could not be fixed in an adequate position on the nose. The earliest representation is found on a fresco painted in 1352 by Tomaso di Modena in the capitol hall of San Nicoló church in Treviso, Italy [11].

In Strossmayer's Gallery of Ancient Masters in Zagreb the painting 'Adulteress before Christ' by Lodovico Mazzolino (c.1480–after 1528) is kept. One of the figures, a Scribe or Pharisee, holds a pair of spectacles on his nose and wears a spectacle case attached to his belt (Fig. 3). The shape of the case itself and the way he holds his spectacles proves that they were of the earliest type, i.e., rivet spectacles [12].

From the beginning, spectacles were rare and valuable objects that could not be fixed permanently on one's face. They had to be safely kept and protected. For this purpose a pear-shaped flat spectacle case was developed. The upper third of the case could be opened to receive the folded spectacles. Spectacle cases were made of iron, copper or bronze sheets, wood, and later of cardboard. Some spectacle cases were even made of silver. Tied to a string, the case was carried attached to the waistbelt. Spectacle cases are seen on paintings from the second half of the 15th century. Examples are found on the paintings of St. Bernardine of Siena by B. Vivarini (c.1430–c.1499) in the Louvre, Paris, and St. Bernardine of Siena by C. Crivelli (1430/35 – c.1493) in the Accademia in Florence.

In the cathedral church at Krk (on the island of Krk) there is the gothic silver altar-piece, made in 1477 by Venetian master Paul Koler and donated by the Croatian noble family Frankopan. Among the numerous saints shown, the figure of St. Bernadine of Siena is represented with a spectacle case hanging from his belt (Fig. 4).

In the Graphic Cabinet of the Croatian Academy of Sciences and Arts in Zagreb several works of Albrecht Dürer (1471–1528) are kept. Among the

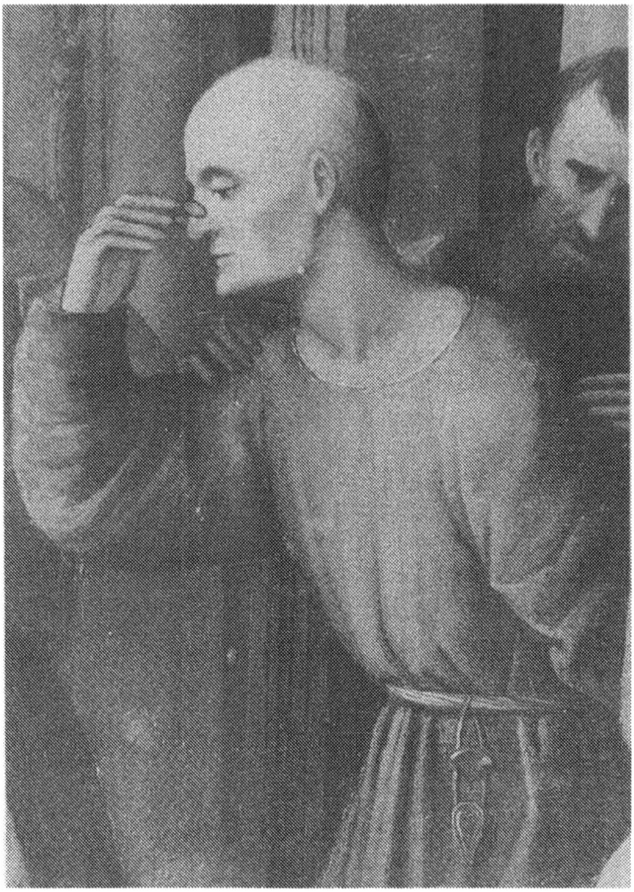

Fig. 3. L. Mazzolino (c.1480–after 1528), 'Adulteress before Christ'. (Detail of the painting, (Strossmayer's Gallery of Ancient Masters, Croatian Academy of Sciences and Arts, Zagreb).

woodcuts of the series The Life of the Virgin (1501–1510/11) there is a scene depicting 'Joachim's offering' (1502/4). One of the priests who refuses a sacrificial lamb offered in the Temple by Joachim, has in one hand a book and in the other the rivet spectacles held in a typical manner in front of his eyes (Fig. 5).

Several written documents from the 16th century deal with spectacles. A pair of spectacles is mentioned in the list of personal belongings of the Venetian official Paul Bolani who died in Trogir in 1511 [13]. By request of the deceased's heir all personal belongings of the late Antun de Benessa were recorded in Dubrovnik on 7 March 1513. Among other things '24 astagi ochiali voti senza li ochiali' (24 empty spectacle cases without spectacles) were noted [14].

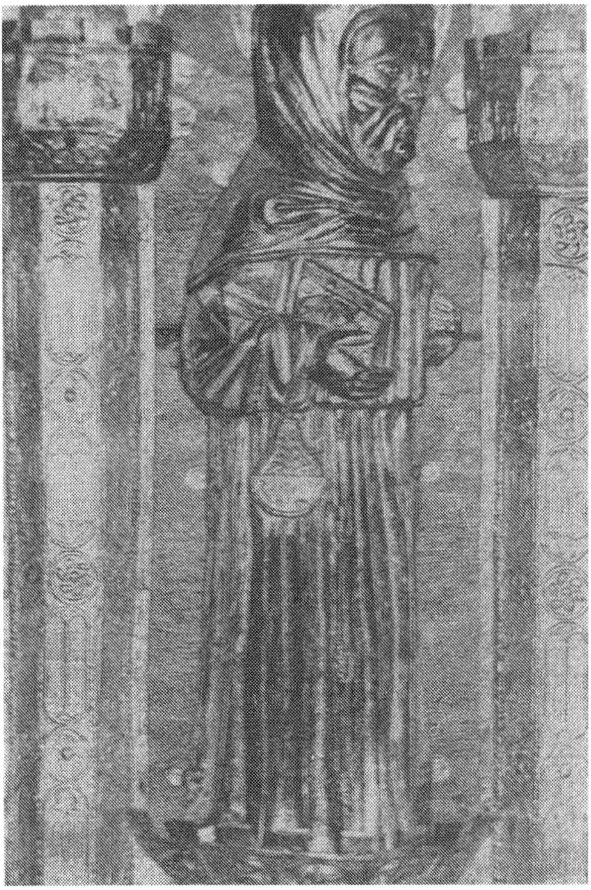

Fig. 4. P. Koler (1477): St. Bernardine of Siena. Ornamented spectacle case hanging from the belt (Detail of the silver alter-piece, Krk Cathedral).

The De Ciprianis family in Trogir has been mentioned since the end of the 12th century. 'Inventarium omnium bonorum mobilum et stabilium quondam domini Joannis de Ciprianis' (Inventory of the complete property of Joannes de Ciprianis), nobleman and owner of a large library, was compiled in 28 August 1528, in Zadar. In the original text under inventory number 27, are listed '...uno par de ochiali cum la sua cassa' (a pair of spectacles with its case) [15].

A similar list of personal belongings of Ilija Lose, who had recently died, was drawn on 29 October 1554, in Dubrovnik. A pair of spectacles was mentioned therein as well ('uno paro de ochiali') [16].

Two documents from the Dubrovnik State Archives, written on 30 December 1563, contain the inventory of the first printer in Belgrade,

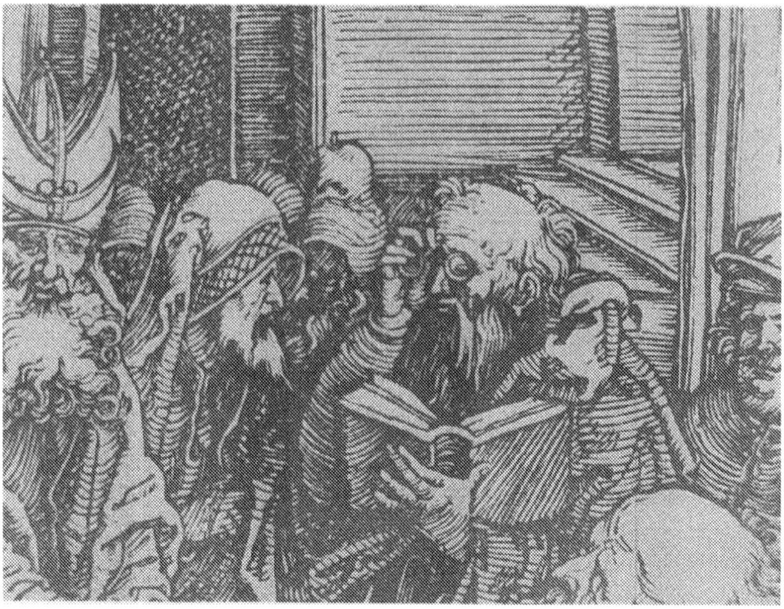

Fig. 5. A. Dürer: Joachim's offering. Priest with rivet spectacles (Detail of the woodcut from 1502/4 Graphic Cabinet of the Croatian Academy of Sciences and Arts, Zagreb).

Trojan Gundulić [17]. Trojan Gundulić was also barber, so that beside his barber's tools, 5 pairs of spectacles are mentioned ('briglie no 2 e briglie No 3').

A portrait of bishop Toma Nigris (c.1450–after 1531) is kept in the Franciscan monastery in Poljud (Split). The bishop was a humanist and organizer of the struggle against the Turkish rule and a prominent and honoured person in his time. The portrait painted in 1527 by Lorenzo Lotto (c.1480–1556) shows the bishop kneeling in prayer with a breviary and a pair of spectacles on a praying desk before him (Fig. 6). Reflected light indicates that the lenses were convex and the spectacles were of the bridge type (Bügelbrille). This type is characterized by framed lenses joined by a firm arc, resembling a tiny bridge. Such spectacles spread fast at the beginning of the 16th century, replacing the heavy, angular and sharp rivet spectacles.

A pair of spectacles from the first half of the 16th century with the remnants of their wooden case was found in the tomb of the patrician family Florio in the Franciscan monastery in Poljud (Split). Spectacles similar to those of bishop Nigris, are kept in the monastery collection. Round lenses were rimmed by a continuous piece of wire, so that the elastic bridge which kept the two lenses together also held the spectacles firmly on the nose. Lenses were made of good quality glass, they were biconvex with a power of + 4.0 and + 4.25 diopters (Fig. 7).

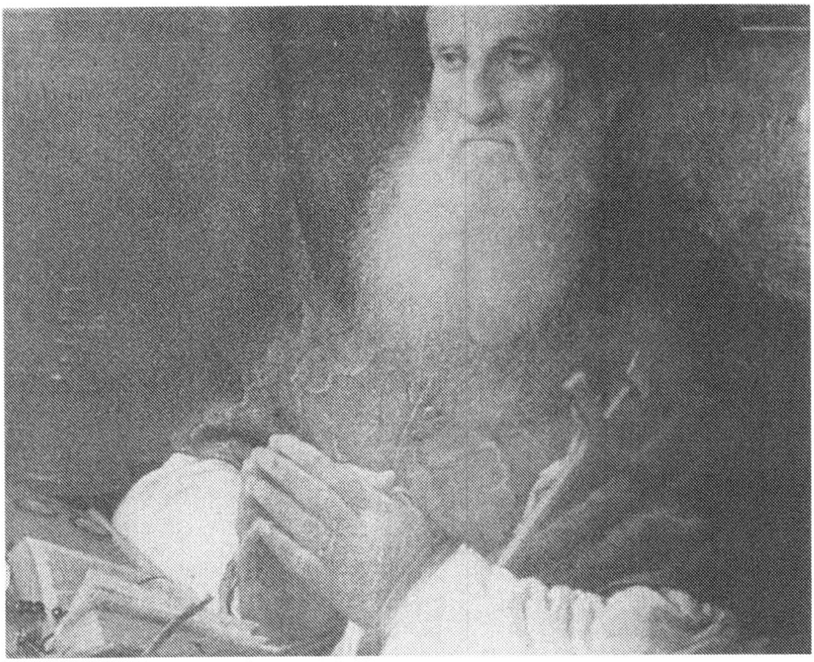

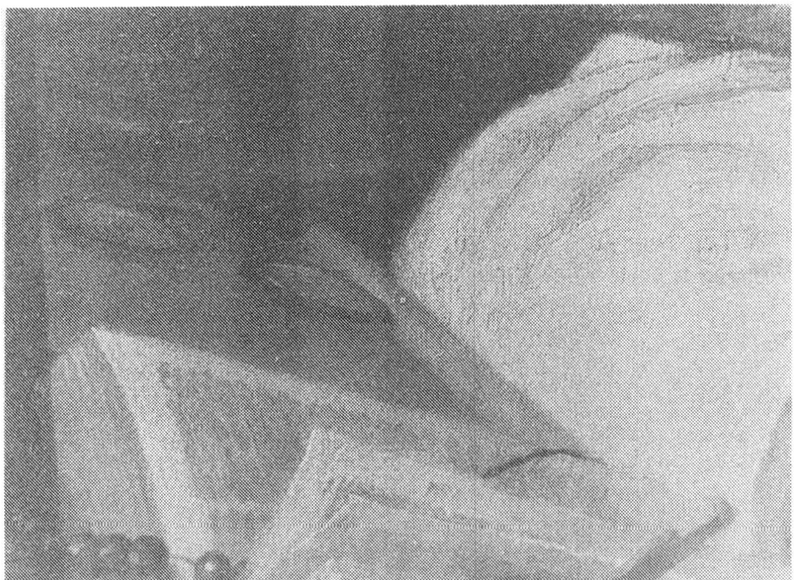

Fig. 6. L. Lotto: Bishop Toma Nigris (Detail of the portrait from 1527, Franciscan monastery, Poljud, Split).

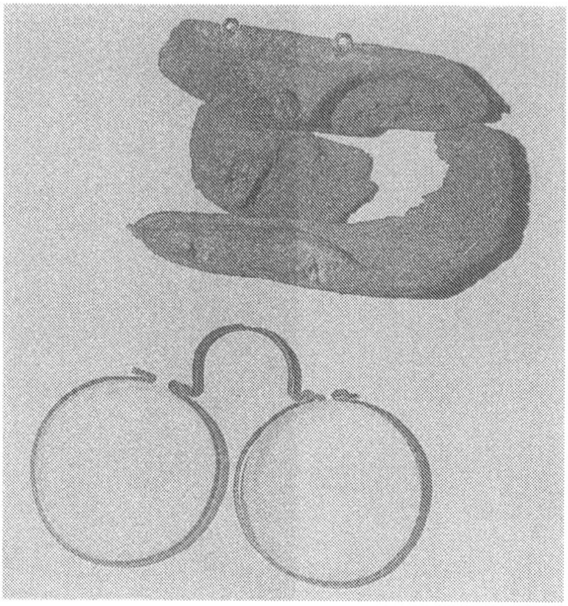

Fig. 7. Spectacles from the Florio family tomb, 16th century (Franciscan monastery collection, Poljud, Split).

Between 1967 and 1969, the remains of a ship probably sailing from Venice and of the goods , were salvaged from the bottom of the sea near Gnalić, a small island south-east of the island of Pašman. The year of shipwreck (after 1582) is confirmed by the date cast in one of the ship's guns [18]. The shipwreck is a hydroarcheological site of major importance, abundant in various material remains and goods which are presently part of the Archaeological collections in Biograd-on-Sea and in the National Museum in Zadar.

Some 20 wooden boxes, half of them damaged, were found packed together with rolls of brass wire and metal sheets. The boxes were made for the transport of spectacles and according to their number, the ship must have carried approximately 300 pairs of spectacles. The boxes were made of thin pieces of board, bent and glued together (like modern matchboxes). Dimensions of one of the better preserved boxes are 100 × 65 × 60 mm. Some 20 spectacles could be packed into a large box, and 10 into a smaller one (S. Petricioli, personal communication).

These spectacles were of the leather-framed type (Lederbrillen) [19]. Round lenses were fitted into a frame made of 5–6 lamellas of pressed leather. The rims of the lenses were joined by a somewhat wider and more massive bridge, that still has the lines impressed into the leather. The leather rim around the lens is 2.5–3.0 mm wide, and 3 mm thick. In smaller and bigger models of spectacles the bridge is 5 and 6 mm wide, respectively.

Dimensions of the large spectacles are 85 × 40 mm, distance between the centres of the lenses is ca. 50 mm, the outer frame diameter is ca. 36 mm, and the inner frame diameter is ca. 32 mm. Dimensions of the smaller type spectacles are 78 × 38–40 mm, distance between the centres of the lenses is ca. 44 mm, the outer frame diameter is ca. 34 mm, and the inner diameter is ca. 28–29 mm. The slit for the nose is 8–9 mm wide.

Dimensions of the boxes and spectacle frames indicate that the spectacles were made in two different sizes (Fig. 8), supposedly for men and for women. Since the round lenses, 30 mm in diameter, were completely opaque and of pearly-green-brownish-black colour, brittle, laminated like mica, their refractive power had to be determined spherometrically. Some of the better preserved lenses had a refractive power of + 3.0 to + 3.5 Diopters.

Other glass objects found on the shipwreck (window panes, wine glasses, etc.) remained transparent and almost unchanged in comparison with the lenses. This glass was obviously of a different composition. Glass analysis performed in the institute for silicate chemistry and technology in Zagreb, revealed indeed a difference in the chemical composition [20].

Transparent and well-preserved glass objects respond to the so-called sodium glass characteristic for Venetian glass manufacture. The lenses, however, were made of potassium glass which was produced in central and northern Europe, mainly in Germany.

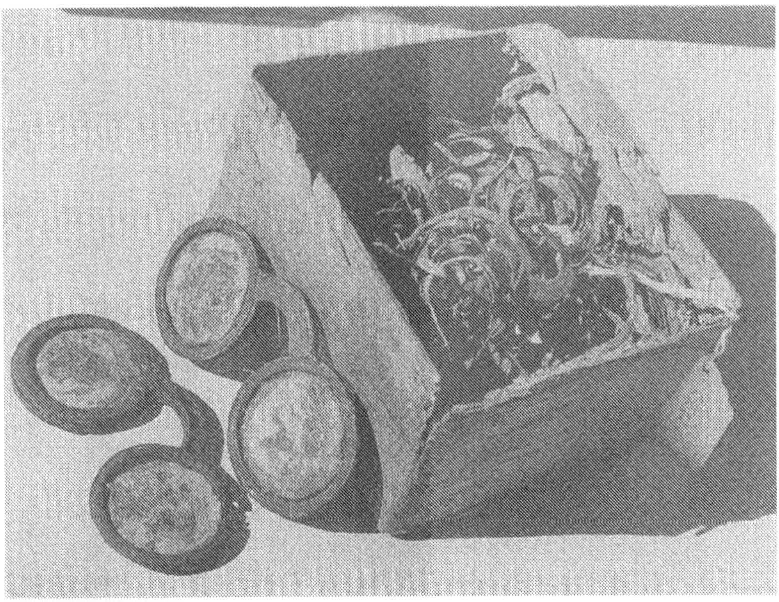

Fig. 8. Leather spectacles and a wooden box in which they were packed, 16th century (National Museum, Zadar).

Considering the fact that the boxes containing spectacles were packed together with brass wire rolls, metal sheets and pins, which came mainly from central Germany, it is assumed that the spectacles were produced in Nürnberg. At that time this town was a leading center of the manufacture of brass, needles and spectacles. It is unlikely that the lenses were produced in Venice from which the other glass objects came.

At the beginning of the 17th century Marko Antun de Dominis (1560–1624), archbishop of Split, philosopher, mathematician and physicist, wrote a book titled 'De radiis visus et lucis in vitris perspectivis et iride'. The book was published in Venice in 1611, and deals with spectacles for the correction of senile (presbyopic) vision – vitrum senile, vitrum convexum seu lenticulare – which he used himself. He also mentioned spectacles for the

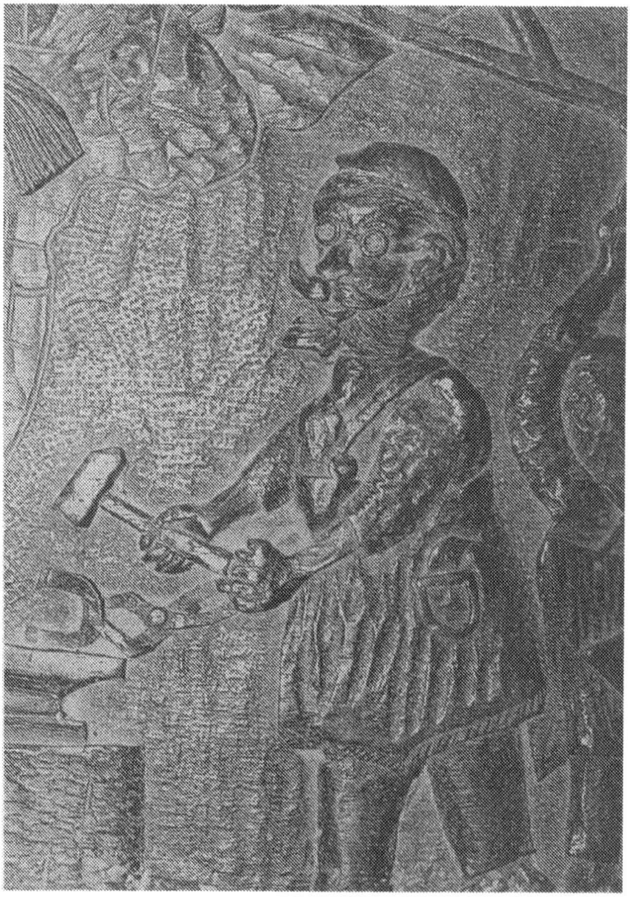

Fig. 9. Blacksmith with spectacles. Lid of the carved wooden guild's box, 17th century (Town Museum, Varaždin).

correction of 'debile vision' (shortsightedness) – vitra excavata, concava. He did not provide, though, a Croatian translation of these terms [21].

Croatian and Latin words for spectacles, spectacle case, and even for the profession of 'ocularius faber' (optician), are found in dictionaries from the 17th century on [22–24].

A check of the blacksmith's guild from the second half of the 17th century is kept in the Town Museum in Varaždin. It is made of brown oak and elaborately carved. The figure of a bearded blacksmith with eyeglasses is seen on the lid [25]. (Fig. 9). The lenses are round with wide frames joined with an arc. These spectacles are the first ones depicted with two side-pieces extending over the ears. They can be considered as spectacles in the modern sense of the word (Ohrenbrille), with round lenses and a characteristic

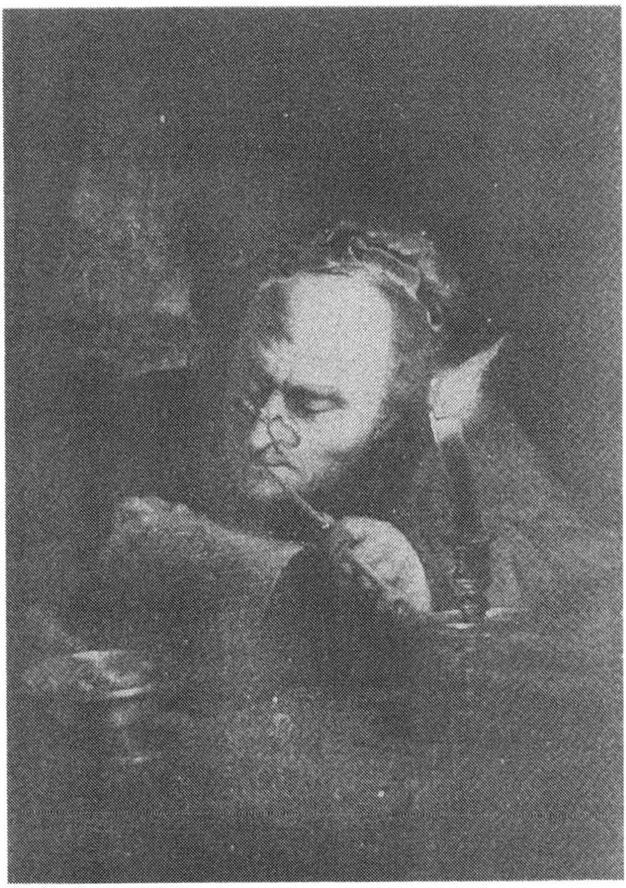

Fig. 10. J. Verkolje (1650–1693): A reading men. Klemmer clip spectacles. (Painting in Mimara Museum, ATM 713, Zagreb–Foto: N.Ćaće).

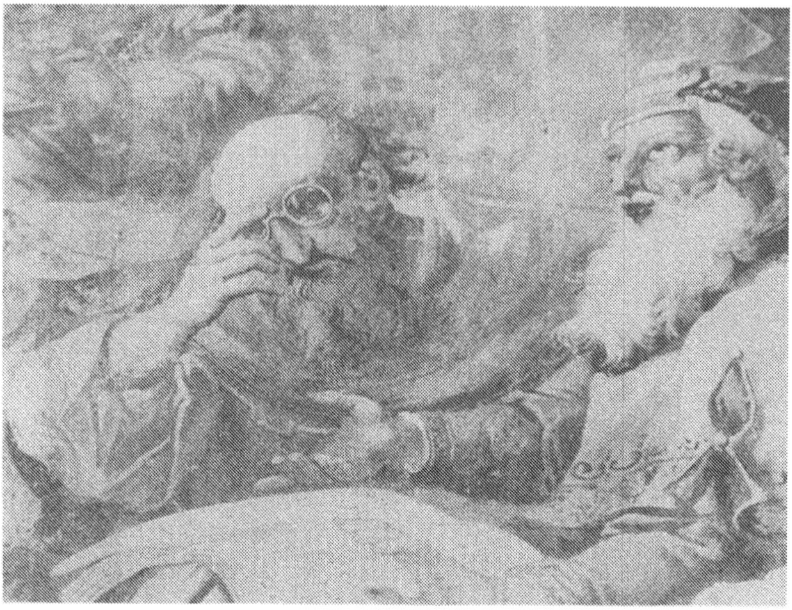

Fig. 11. I. Ranger: Scribe with spectacles. Detail of the fresco 'Twelve-year-old Jesus in the Temple', 1742 (Monastery St. Mary's church, Lepoglava).

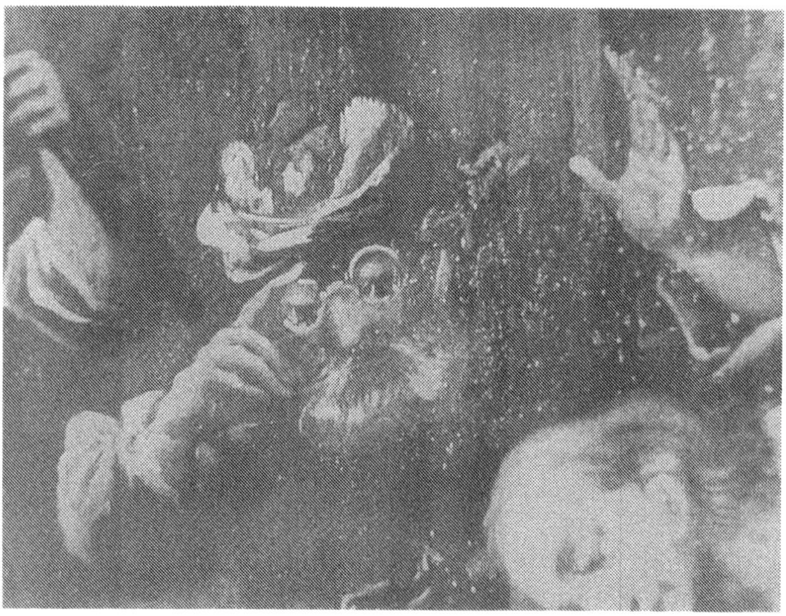

Fig. 12. I. Ranger: 'Adulteress before Christ'. Pale horn or bone spectacles of bridge type (Detail of painted back of the choice stalls from 1743, St. Mary's church, Lepoglava).

17th-century frame. It is still not clear whether they were intended as presbyopic or protective spectacles.

In the Mimara Museum in Zagreb in the painting 'A reading man' by Dutch painter Jan Verkolje (1650–1693) is kept. In the picture, painted in characteristic chiaroscuro, a man reading by candle light uses Klemmer clip (nose-pinching) spectacles, very popular in the seventeenth century (Fig. 10). Round-eye lenses were mounted in specially shaped metal wire rim and joined by a bow spring. Another example of a pince-nez is shown on the painting 'Old reading women' (c.1629) by the famous Dutch master Rembrandt (1609–1669) [26].

Ivan Ranger (1700–1753), master of Croatian baroque painting, worked in Lepoglava, the center of Pauline order in Croatia and the cultural and artistic center of his time. In 1742, he painted illusionistic frescoes of high artistic quality in the monastery church of St. Mary's. [27]. The scene

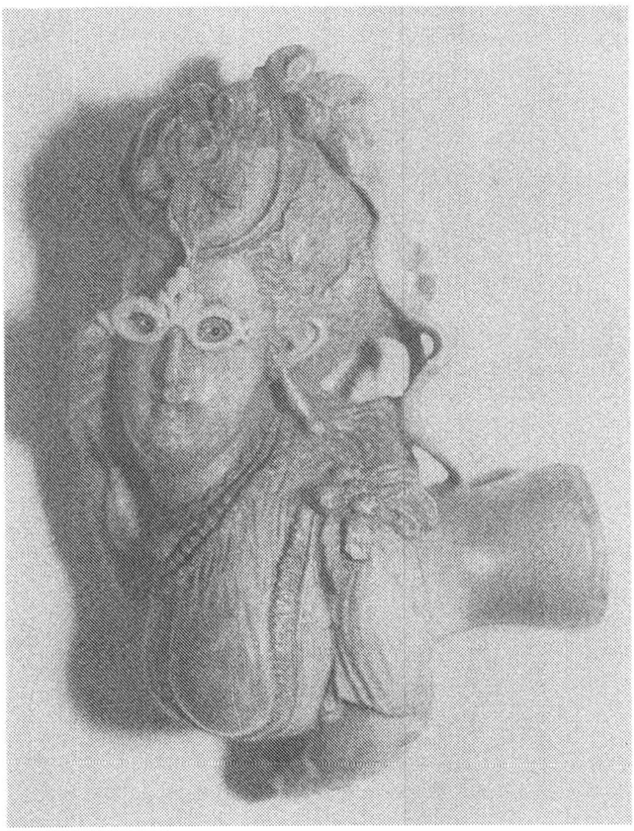

Fig. 13. Fashion spectacles made of ivory. Artistic carved pipe-bowl, 18/19th century (Town Museum, Varaždin).

'Twelve-year old Jesus in the Temple' is painted on the right-hand wall of the church sanctuary. One of the Scribes is engrossed in a book, and holds his spectacles with one hand. They have round lenses, fine, firm, light-coloured frames and ornamented bridges (Fig. 11). The painting probably represents the pale, horn-framed bridge spectacles (Bügelbrille).

In 1743, the Pauline monk Ivan Ranger and his coworkers painted the backs of the choir stalls in the St. Mary's church in Leolglava. Among the depicted themes on Jesus' public activity and miracles there is a painting 'A woman caught in adultery and Jesus' (John 8,2–11). One of the Pharisees or Scribes looks at the words written on the ground by Jesus. He holds a bridge spectacles with big round lenses rimmed in a massive light-coloured frame, probably made of horn or bone (Fig. 12).

In the official documents of the Varaždin township dating from 1786. Haller, 'vitriarius et oculista', is mentioned [28].

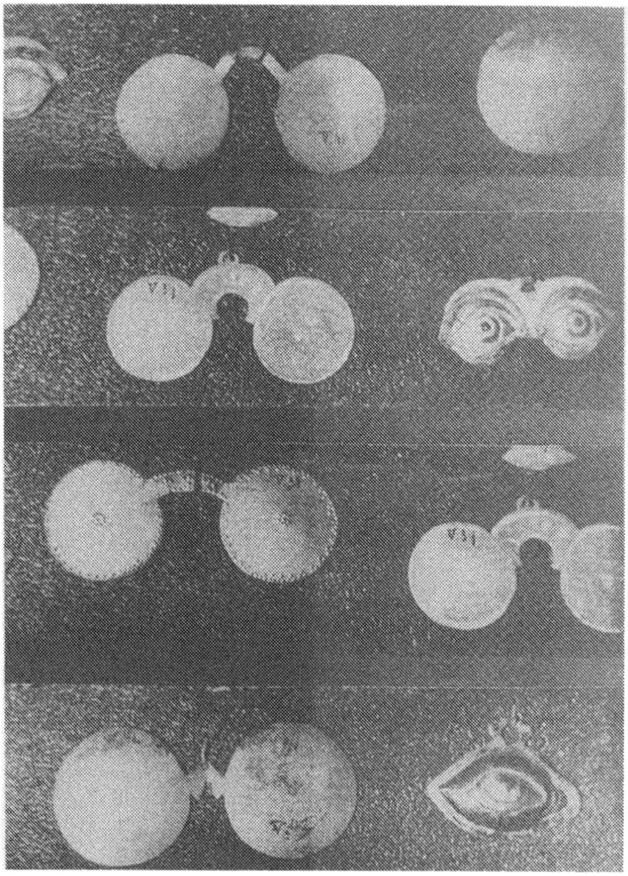

Fig. 14. Votive silver spectacles, 18/19th (Diocesan Museum, Zagreb).

Spectacles as a fashion item are represented as detail of an artistic carved pipe-bowl in wood (Fig. 13). The pipe-bowl, sculpted as the bust of the coquette lady (from the second half of eighteenth century) is kept in the town Museum in Varaždin. Oval lenses are held by a small ring-shaped handle; the bridge is very finely ornamented. The white frame indicates the fashion of spectacles made of ivory or bone.

The Diocesan museum in Zabreb exhibits votive spectacles. These are of the bridge type and of normal size (Fig. 14), and made of partly ornamented

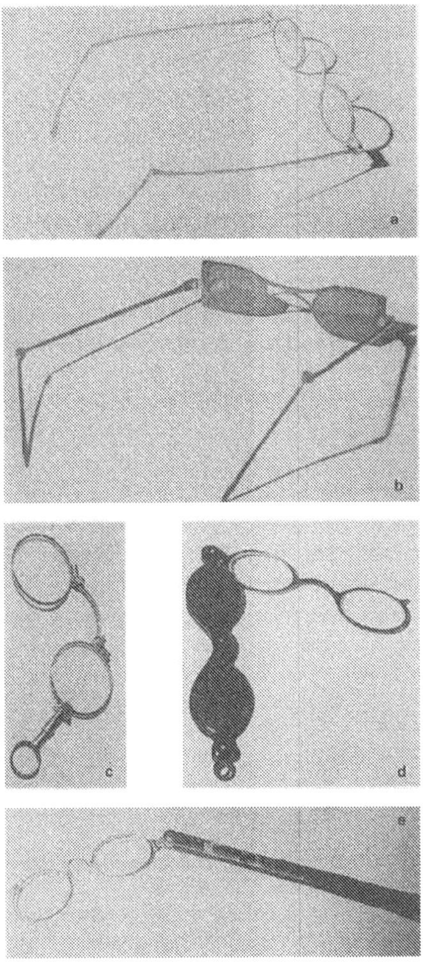

Fig. 15. Nineteenth and early twentieth-century spectacles. Town Museum Samobor. (From top to bottom): (a) Brass spectacles with turn-pin side. First half of 19th c.; (b) Protective green glass spectacles of the French style. First half of 19th c.; (c) Spring semi-lorgnette, early 20th c.; (d) Tortoise-shell lorgnette, early 20th c.; (e) Long-handled tortoise-shell lorgnette with nickled frame. From the turn of the century.

silver plates. Goldsmiths' marks indicate that they originate from the second half of the 18th century and the first half of the 19th century [29].

Several nineteenth century and early twentieth-century spectacles are kept in the Town Museum of Samobor (Fig. 15). Small round-eye brass spectacles with turn-pin side Ayscough-type (double-fold sides) date from c. 1820. Light protective green glass spectacles of the 'French style' date probably from the first half of nineteenth-century. Semi-oval lenses with K-bridge frames are made of tortoise-shell with metal turn-pin side Taylor-type. The nickled and long-handled tortoise-shell lorgnette (so called glove or dowager-duchess type) dates from the turn of this century. Both, spring semi-lorgnette made of nickel and oval-lensed shell lorgnette, date from the early twentieth century [30].

Studying the history of spectacles and comparing various historical sources dealing with the development of spectacles in the world and in Croatia, it can be concluded that this important civilizational achievement was used in Croatia very early in its history. Close vicinity of northern Italy, the native land of spectacles, certainly influenced such a course of events.

Strong ties linked Croatia to European cultural circles. Transfer of spiritual and material goods between the eastern and western Adriatic coast and vice versa, enabled Croatia to be one of the few nations which enjoyed the benefits of spectacles already in the first hundred years of their history.

Acknowledgements

A record of spectacles in the Historical Archives in Zadar was kindly called to my attention by Prof. Dr. Ivo Petricioli, Zadar. For the information about spectacles in the Historical Archives in Dubrovnik I am much obliged to Prof. Ivo Ficović from the Historical Archives of that city.

References

1. Magnifica Comunita di Zara, No. 120. Inventari 1325–1493, Busta Ia, Fasciculo I° (1–120).
2. Traljić MS. Vodeni znakovi u dokumentima i rukopisma samostana Svete Marije u Zadru. Zafar: Radovi Instituta JAZU, 1967; 13–14: 167–74.
3. Greeff R. Die ältesten Formen der Brillenfassungen. Klin Mbl Augenheilkd 1934; 93: 94–9.
4. Briquet CM. Les Filigranes. Dictionnaire historique des Marques du Papier, dès leur apparition vers 1282 jusqu'en 1600, avec 39 figures dans le texte et 16112 fac-similis de filigranes. 3. Tom. Paris: A. Picarde et fils, 1907.
5. Mošin AV, Traljić S. Vodeni znakovi XIII i XIV vijeka. Tom I. Zagreb: Historijski institut JAZU, 1957: 85–119.
6. Historical Archives in Dubrovnik. Lamenta de intus, vol. 12. Fol. 194. See also: Han V. Arhivske vesti o staklu u Dubrovniku iz XIV i prve polovine XV veka. Zbornik 15. Beograd: Muzej primenjene umetnosti, 1971: 57.

7. Historical Archives in Dubrovnik. Diversa notarie. Vol. 37. Fol. 62v–65r.
8. Historical Archives in Dubrovnik. Diversa Cancellarie. Vol. 82. Fol. 78.
9. Grubenbecher H, Appuhn H. Kloster Wienhausen. Hamburg: H. Ellermann, 1955. See also: Appuhn H. Kloster Wienhausen. Der Fund vom Nonnenchor. Bd. IV, Verl. Kloster Wienhausen, 1973.
10. Greeff R. Die historische Entwicklung der Brille (Eine Anleitung zum Verständnis der Brillenausstellung in dem Heidelberger Museum). Bericht DOG 1913; 39: 419–51.
11. Schmitz EH. Die Sehhilfe im Wandel der Jahrhunderte. Stuttgart: Süddeutsche Optiker-Zeitung Verlag, 1961: 13–86.
12. Greeff R. Die älteste Brillendarstellung auf einem Tafelbild (anno 1404). Arch Augenheilkd 1925; 96: 65–71.
13. Grmak MD. Naočari, Povijest. In: Medicinska Enciklopedija. Zagreb: Jugoslavenski leksikografski zavod, 1963, 7: 174–76.
14. Historical Archives in Dubrovnik. Diversa Cancellaire. Vol. 109. Fol. 233r–v.
15. Miscelanea II–IV. Zadar: Državni arhiv Zadar, 1950–1952: 54–63.
16. Historical Archives in Dubrovnik. Diversa notarie. Vol. 113. Fol. 250v.
17. Kesterčanek F. Inventar prvog beogradskog tiskara Trojana Gundulića. Anali historijskog instituta u Dubrovniku 1952; 1: 197–206.
18. Petricioli I. Sidra i topovi. Vrulje 1970; 1: 9–15.
19. von Pflugk A. Lederbrillen. Zschr. Ophthalmol Optik 1928; 16: 2–10.
20. Kuzmek V. Laslo R. Staklos broda potonulog kod otočića Gnalić. Emajl-keramika-staklo 1971; 7: 30–37.
21. Dugački V. M.A. Dominis i problemi vida. In: Zbornik radova o M.A. Dominisu i znanstvenoj prošlosti otoka Raba. Zagreb: Skupština općine Rab, 1976: 85–91.
22. Jacobus Micalia. Thesaurus lingue Illyricae sive Dictionarium Illyricum in quo verba italicae et latine reduntur. Laureti: Apud Paulum & JO. Baptistam Seraphinum, 1649.
23. Joannis Bellosztenecz. Gazophylacium seu Latino-Illyricorum onomatum aerarium. Zagrabiae: Typis Joannis Bapt. Weitz, 1740.
24. Andrea Jambressich. Lexicon latinus interpretatione illyrica, germanica et hungarica locuplex, in usum potissimum studiosae juventutis digestum. Zagrabiae: 1742.
25. Štajduhar J. Prikaz naočala na varaždinskoj cehovskoj škrinji iz XVI. stoljeća. In: Iz hrvatske medicinske prošlosti, Snomen knjiga ZLH. Zagreg: Zbor liječnika Hrvatske, 1954: 202–04.
26. Schitz EH. Die Sehhilfe im Wandel der Jahrhunderte. Stuttgart: Verlag Süddeutsche Optikerzeitung, 1961: 66–75.
27. Mirković M. Ivan Krstitelj Ranger i pavlinsko slikarstvo. In: Kultura pavlina u Hrvatskoj 1244–1786. Zagreb: Globus, 1989: 127–163, 430–433.
28. Archives of Croatia, Zagreb, Documents of Varaždin township 196/1786.
29. Bach I. Zlatarski radovi u riznici zagrebačke katedrale sa žigovima mariborskih i zagrebačkih majstora 18. st. Tkalčićev zbornik II. Zagreb, 1958.
30. Davidson DC. Spectacles, Lorgnettes and Monocles. Aylesbury (Bucks): Shire Publications, 1989: 16–21.

Address for correspondence: Prof. Dr. Vjekoslav Dorn, University Eye Clinic, Kišpatićeva 12, 41000 Zagreb, Croatia
Phone: (041) 233–233, ext. 403.

Documenta Ophthalmologica **86**: 191–202, 1994.

Pissarro, dacryocystitis, and the development of modern lacrimal surgery

JAMES G. RAVIN
The Eye Center of Toledo, Toledo, Ohio, USA

Key words: History of ophthalmology, Medicine and the arts, Lacrimal surgery

Abstract. The co-founder of French Impressionism, Camille Pissarro, suffered from chronic dacryocystitis for at least fifteen years. This kept him from working for long periods of time, and when he was able to work, influenced his method of painting. Pissarro just missed the modern period of lacrimal surgery, and was treated by conservative methods.

Introduction

Pissarro, the elder statesman of French Impressionism had a long artistic career. Born in 1830, he died in 1903 at the age of 73. He was, with Claude Monet, a founder and leader of the French Impressionist movement. He was also a colleague and friend of Degas, Renoir, Seurat, Cassatt, and Van Gogh. Pissarro was the only member of the Impressionist group to exhibit at every one of their shows, from 1874 until 1876. His productivity during the last 15 years of his life was hampered by recurrent infections around his right eye. These problems troubled him greatly, and necessitated multiple visits to his ophthalmologist in Paris for care. When Pissarro was able to work, the ocular problems influenced his method of painting.

The history of Pissarro's malady is interesting for the light it sheds on a major artist's method of adjusting to adversity. The story also provides a view of one aspect of the history of medical care in the late 19th century, with interesting comparisons to medical care today.

This artist was an ardent follower of homeopathic therapy. He acquired his mother's faith in homeopathy during a severe illness she had suffered many years earlier. Pissarro frequently consulted a book of remedies that he kept at home, and often mailed advice to his children after they had grown and moved away.

Pissarro found an ophthalmologist who utilized homeopathic therapy in Daniel Parenteau, MD (1842–c.1935). Parenteau was trained in traditional allopathic medicine, but employed homeopathic medications. Although he advocated homeopathic drugs, he was not opposed to surgery. He was a member of the French Ophthalmologic Society from

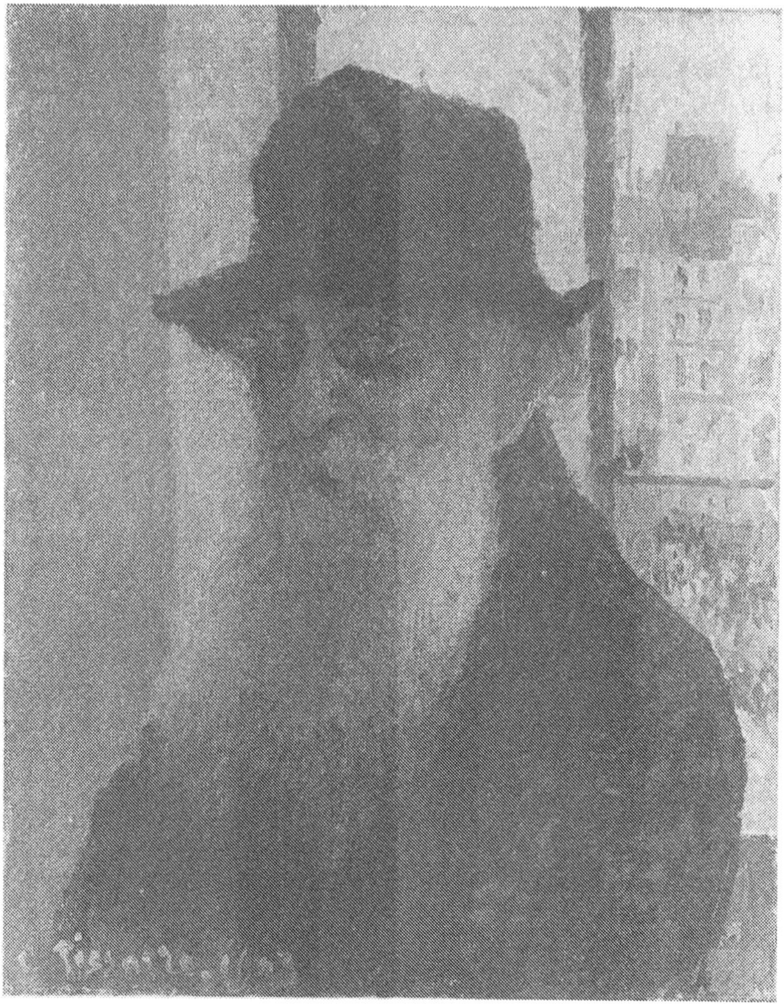

Fig. 1. Pissarro. Self-Portrait. Oil on canvas, 1903. $16\frac{1}{2} \times 18\frac{1}{8}$ inches. London, Tate Gallery.

1884 through 1926.[1] The membership rolls of the Homeopathic Medical Society of France list his name from 1900 through 1935, and he was president of that society in 1901 and 1902.[2] Parenteau published occasionally in the homeopathic literature, but more often in ophthalmologic medical publications. He wrote three books; *Leçons de Clinique Ophtalmologique*,[3] *Education de l'oeil et son hygiène*,[4] and *Thérapeutique homéopathique en ophtalmologie*.[5]

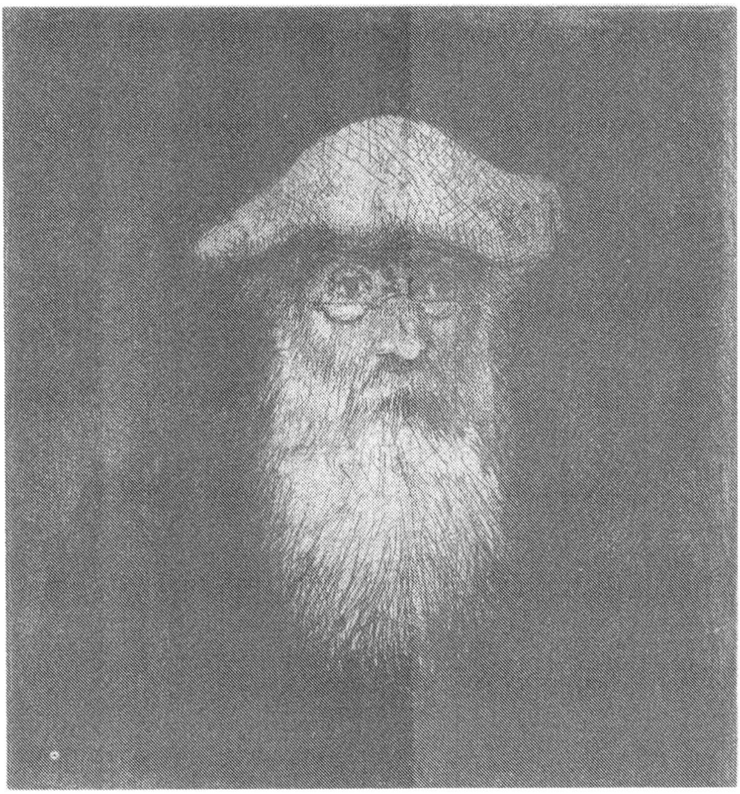

Fig. 2. Pissarro. Self-Portrait. Etching on zinc, 1890–91. $7\frac{1}{4} \times 7\frac{3}{8}$ inches. Boston Public Library.

Ocular problems

Pissarro suffered from chronic infection of the tear sac with fistula formation during the last fifteen years of his life. The date he first developed this is not known, but it certainly was present by 1889, when he described the results of a visit to his ophthalmologist. In May 1889 Parenteau found Pissarro's right nasal lacrimal duct was blocked. He probed the passages and found a bony obstruction. He told the artist that attempting to force a probe through the blocked area could create disastrous complications. Instead, he prescribed a homeopathic medication, Aurum, in the hope that it would allow the tissues around the bone to heal. He told Pissarro healing would take at

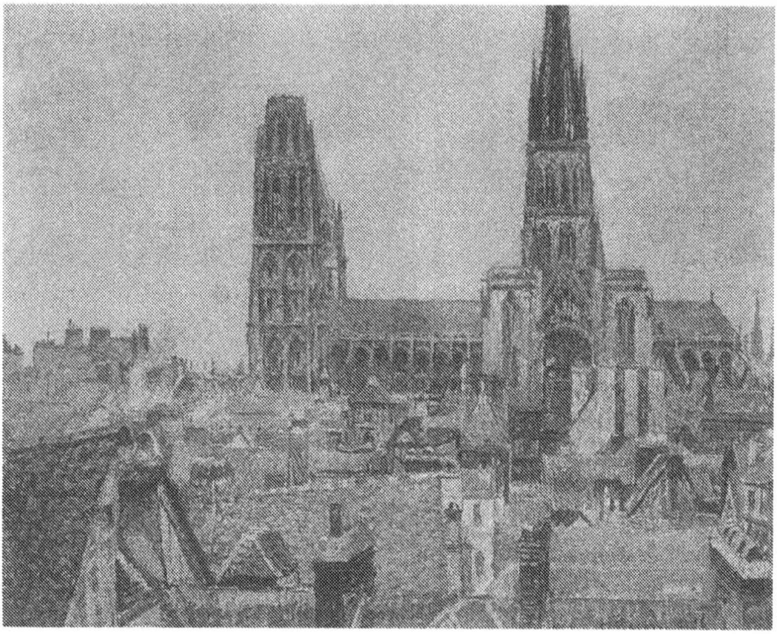

Fig. 3. Pissarro. The Roofs of Old Rouen. Oil on canvas, 1896. $28\frac{1}{2} \times 36$ inches. Toledo Museum of Art.

least six months, and that he should take care to 'avoid wind and dust, and wash the eye immediately with boric acid should anything get in it.' Pissarro noted 'all that is hardly easy for a painter who ought to face the elements.'[6]

Seven weeks later Pissarro reported 'Dr. Parenteau found that the lacrimal sac has flattened out but swelling persists near the lacrimal canal, at the inner corner of the eye. Because of this, I have to keep a dressing over my eye for at least a month . . . If after a month things have not improved, it will be necessary to make a small incision in the swollen area to allow the tissues to heal properly, so that tears can flow normally.'[7]

Nearly a year and a half later, in January 1891, Pissarro wrote his son Lucien 'I am very troubled at this moment. My eye has been irritated by the intense cold weather and is swollen. It is threatening to turn into an abscess. I must see Dr. Parenteau.'[8] Later that month, he reported, 'Parenteau has found me much better . . . I must keep a bandage over the eye for ten more days. This is very annoying.'[9] He continued 'I shall try to work with one eye. Degas does it and gets good results.'[10]

In March 1891, Pissarro optimistically wrote Lucien 'My eye is doing well. I saw Parenteau, who was very happy with the result. He advised me to put a patch over the eye in bad weather. In two weeks, if things are the same, if the walls of the tear sac come together, I will be cured. Things have gone well up till now. For a month I have not had any swelling.'[11] But a month

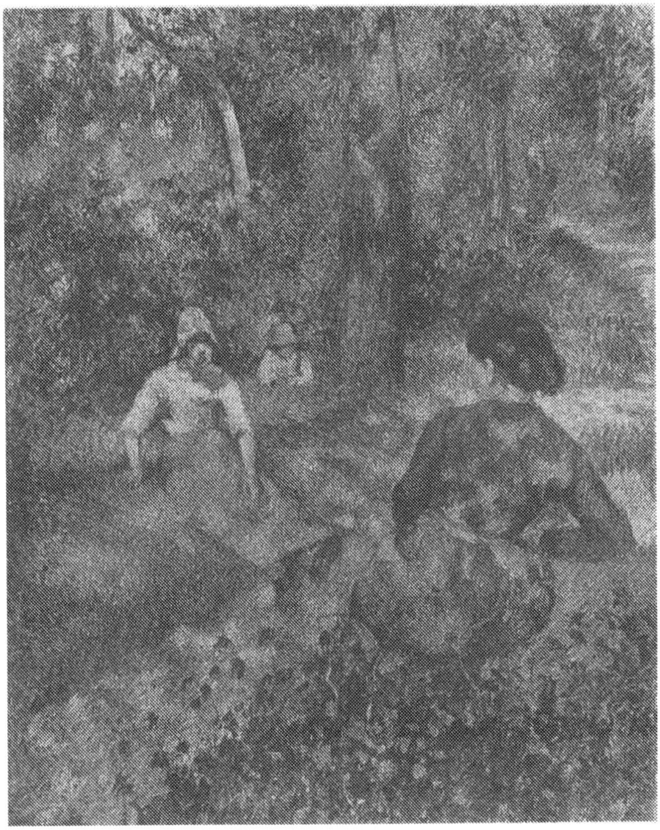

Fig. 4. Pissarro. Peasants Resting. Oil on canvas, 1881. $32 \times 25\frac{3}{4}$ inches. Toledo Museum of Art.

later he wrote 'A new abscess has developed. I am forced to suspend all work.'[12] He returned to Paris, and saw Parenteau, who probably drained the area again. Two days later Pissarro noted that the abscess was nearly gone.[13]

Second and third opinions

Pissarro sought advice from other doctors. One young physician told him 'destruction of the sac was not a good answer to his problem, since tears would continue to flow copiously.' For a painter, this could be a serious difficulty that could prevent him from working. This doctor advised him 'the only thing to do is to try to find the passage through bone into the nose. Break through the bone into the nose, and use sounds of progressively larger sizes to maintain the opening, or else remove the bone which blocks the canal and obstructs the flow of tears.' Pissarro met an older physician who told him 'he had the same problem as I, and forty years earlier he had his first symptoms. This doctor's friends and colleagues advised surgery, but he declined, and the sac closed itself off. He lived that way for forty years without difficulty, except for a bit of tearing, which was tolerable. He was lucky. However, this doctor told me that the sac does not ever atrophy totally and that further abscesses could still form.'[14] Pissarro then questioned Parenteau at greater length about these two alternatives, surgery versus medical therapy. At age sixty, Pissarro was no longer young, and was afraid of operative complications. He felt Parenteau had managed his case well, and concluded he should continue with him.

Treatment in the late 19th century

Pissarro's consultants were aware of the level of understanding of lacrimal disease at the time. Lacrimal problems were a popular topic in France in 1891. That year, in the *Archives d'Ophtalmologie*, Albert Terson summarized the experience of the Hotel Dieu Hospital, in Paris. His 19 page article was entitled 'On Destruction of the Sac with Thermocautery and its Total Destruction in Fistulas and Refractory Lacrimal Tumors.'[15] In the *Bulletin and Memoirs of the French Ophthalmological Society*, Alfred Terson (Albert's father) published an exhaustive 34 page 'Report on Treatment of Afflictions of the Lacrimal Passages'[16] This report included discussion by virtually every important contemporary French ophthalmologist, including Trousseau, Parinaud, de Wecker, Chibret, Galejowski, Motais, Panas, Javal, and Kalt.

Unfortunately for Pissarro, he never met the Italian surgeon, Toti, who developed modern lacrimal surgery during Pissarro's lifetime. In 1904, the year following the artist's death, Toti published his method of dacryocystorhinostomy.[17] Toti approached the lacrimal sac through the skin, excised the inner wall of the sac, and chiselled through bone into the nose. He then excised the adjacent nasal mucosa, and closed the skin. He applied a pressure dressing to allow the edges of the lacrimal sac and nasal mucosa to be in contact with each other.

Prior to the development of modern lacrimal surgery, two methods of treating dacryocystitis existed, dacryocystectomy and probing by Bowman's technique. Excision of the sac gave less than ideal results. If any mucosa was left behind, continual suppuration and fistula formation were nearly guaranteed. Removal of the sac destroyed the pathway for tears to the nose, and resulted in constant tearing. Bowman's method of probing, introduced in 1857, involved probing the lacrimal drainage system with sounds of progressively larger and larger diameter.[18] False passages were common which could create cellulitis or further scarring.

On May 7, 1891, Pissarro wrote his son Lucien 'Parenteau has found my status exceptionally good. In fact, in all usual cases of my type, the practice is to operate to make an opening into the nose, so the tears can flow normally. But it appears that in my case, this procedure would be useless. The tears would not follow the normal pathway because the abscess had created passages in abnormal directions. According to him, there is only one thing to do, to obliterate the tear sac. Parenteau told me that there was no other way. There was evidently some disadvantages, but other methods would have even more. Among the complications of this operation are the tendency of the eye to become inflamed and blurry vision. I spoke about this with Dr. de Bellio, who told me he was not concerned about excessive tearing, that Parenteau was correct. But I will have to take great care against getting matter in the eye. For the moment Parenteau had injected the area with silver nitrate, to close off the abnormal passageways created by the abscess and to destroy the sac, while waiting to see if another abscess will form. For the time being , he is allowing the inflammation to destroy the sac. I am now in remission. I will probably have abscesses less frequently in the future, and this will allow me to work a little bit. Besides, I am getting used to the idea of having only one eye for working. This is much better than having none at all.'[19]

As a typical parent, Pissarro finished his letter to his son by giving him advice on taking care of himself. 'You told me you have a bad cold. Take care of yourself. Do not neglect yourself, because so-called minor problems can become very serious. If you find that your nose if often blocked, see an eye doctor. If I had known Parenteau earlier, I would not have had my problem. The same thing can happen to you, considering the shape of your nose.'

Pissarro's Problem Smoldered Along

Three months later, in July 1891, he wrote his son again. 'I have really not had good luck, but I am being patient. The eye problem has caused me much concern. I saw Parenteau yesterday. The abscess has caused some inflammation, which is all right, and will still permit a minor procedure to be done today. This will be a small incision to enlarge the existing opening [canaliculus] a bit, then cautery to close off the sac and abnormal channels formed by the discharge. I hope it will not take long. The only thing to fear is erysipelas, which can prevent the operation from being successful. I am taking large doses of quinine as a preventive measure. I hope to be rid of my problem for a long time. But to be sure of a cure, it will be necessary to avoid a recurrence for a year or two. The tears must keep the normal passages open so that tears can flow out, carrying away debris or foreign matter. Recently, while I was working in our field, in good weather, I got a bit of dirt in the eye. Two days later an abscess formed and broke through.'[20]

Later, in July 1891, he wrote his son that Parenteau, had enlarged the opening made by the abscess and inserted a linen drain to keep the orifice open until the sac closed itself off. Parenteau permitted him to work indoors without a dressing over the eye, if the windows were kept closed.[21] Things had changed little three months later, in the autumn of 1891. Pissarro wrote Lucien, 'I went to see Parenteau yesterday. He found me very well, only I must take more precautions this winter and on windy days.[22]

A year later the situation was basically the same. He wrote his wife, Julie, 'I returned to Parenteau's. He found me a little better. I must continue the medications for 15 days and continue to take precautions for at least a year. There is nothing more to do but to avoid the effects of humidity . . .'[23]

In the spring of 1893 he wrote his son Lucien again. Parenteau had advised him that if he should have a recurrence, 'not to press on the area around the opening to force out pus.'[24] Parenteau was well informed in this regard. He had published articles on massage about the eye and on ocular infections.[25] Pissarro said he could still wear his eye glasses even if they rested near the area involved. 'Today nothing new has occurred, no suppuration, no inflammation,' he said. 'Without anything new, Parenteau thinks that this could be the end of the problem. I am taking Silicea [a homeopathic medication] in large doses to try to absorb the rest of the discharge, and we will see the result in a few days.'[26] Two days later, Pissarro wrote Lucien 'I have come from Parenteau's. The small opening has closed up from below and a small amount of swelling has spread toward the lacrimal canal, which will be operated in the future. I noticed it this morning and am very afraid of this new finding, but Parenteau was pleased.'[27]

The next day, Pissarro noted 'Parenteau injected the area around the eye with silver nitrate, in order to stimulate inflammation and try to close down the small passages which are full of debris. He thinks that it will be necessary to use a stronger caustic agent. In a few days I will see if this treatment has helped. Your mother is impatient and would like to know the name of this illness. She cannot understand that the doctor cannot cure me through magic.'[28] Shortly thereafter Pissarro noted 'My oculist found me better today. The injection of silver nitrate has done me good. There is hardly any discharge. He replaced the dressing over the eye. I hope that it will continue to do well. I am not suffering at all.'[29]

Pissarro soon wrote his wife, 'I have just come from Parenteau's. I did not want to go too soon because it was Ascension day. He examined me and found me very well. He said, however, it is better to let the tissue grow stronger before doing another minor operation. There is no hurry to close off the small channel. He told me that I can return home to Eragny and come back early next month.'[30] In 1893, he wrote Lucien about his fears of recurrences. 'This morning I had a little discharge, without inflammation of the eye. I am very irritated by it. I hope that this will not prevent the operation from being done' In a postscript to that letter, he wrote 'my eye has been a little bit watery for three or four days, nothing more.'[31]

Two days later, he was pleased, as he wrote 'My doctor cannot perform the minor operation for me since the area had not scarred over . . . I am not happy. I am afraid of the smallest cold, especially here with the abrupt changes in the weather.'[32]

That summer he was more despondent. 'Certainly if I were less an old crock on account of my eye, I would like to come visit you next year. But I am not certain of anything. Parenteau's operation cannot be done. No doubt you will remember his idea was to split the tube which drains the tears. Sadly, as he had feared for a long time, the cartilage of the nose has become mildly inflamed from the abscess. This was enough to produce swelling, which has obstructed the narrow passageway. . . In the meantime I am working indoors when it is windy outside.'[33]

In the autumn of 1893, he wrote Lucien, 'Parenteau's treatment has changed nothing. I am taking a mixture of six homeopathic medications by mouth, prescribed by de Bellio . . . So far, there has been no result . . . I will soon try Sutter's homeopathic method.' The following spring he wrote 'I am still going to Parenteau, who is cauterizing the area around the eye, to eliminate the conjunctivitis and the discharge which reoccurs at the slightest change of the weather.'[34]

During the next few years the problem continued to smolder. He wrote Lucien in 1896: 'Parenteau examined me carefully yesterday. My conjunctivitis was complicated by a small amount of inflammation of the cartilage of the nose, although the eye is somewhat better. This has caused a small amount of whitish discharge every morning. Parenteau assured me that this is not very serious, not a bony infection, and if it were that, the pain would have been very severe.'[35]

A week later he wrote Lucien 'your mother has been very anxious and came to Paris to see Parenteau, who reassured her. Certainly I am better, but things are tedious because of the hot weather. We asked Dr. Leon Simon to come see your mother and me in consultation. He treated her for her problem of herpes. Simon found your mother much better and told us that the problem with my eye is not very serious. He prescribed the same medication as Parenteau had, and in response to your mother's question, did I need an operation urgently, he answered no, that was not necessary. It is certainly good that the inflammation of the nasal cartilage is only an inconvenience and not very dangerous. Although an operation can cause unexpected complications, it should not be done if there is a chance of bony destruction, which there is not . . . I am not nervous. What annoys me is to not be able to work outdoors.'[36]

Effect on his painting

Pissarro adapted to the situation. Unable to work outdoors, he would paint indoors looking outward. His city scapes of Rouen and Paris created over the next few years were triumphs. Admittedly some were created in cold weather, but they indicate his method of adapting to adversity. In 1897, Pissarro began a letter to Lucien by prodding him, saying 'You ought to write me from time to time, to exercise your hand a little bit.' He then described his ocular problem: 'I am afraid of complications for my eye. I have gone daily for a dozen days to Parenteau, who has been cauterizing me and has been putting an astringent on the veins of the eye . . . Parenteau gave me silver nitrate drops to put in the eye and on the lids. This is hardly easy. Every morning there is more pus in the eye, so that I dare not venture a trip. Your mother advised me not to leave.' Lucien was about to depart for London, to visit his brother, Titi, who was moribund from tuberculosis. Pissarro wrote 'I hope that you do not go, that you are busy with your work. Aren't you afraid that the London fog will be unfavorable for you? The weather has been exceptional here since you left. Now it is 3:30 and there is a beautiful golden sun outside with a slight mist.'[37]

Lucien's brother, Titi, died four days later, in November 1897, at age 24. Pissarro consoled Lucien. 'I am happy to learn that you have been able to face the disastrous news of the death of our poor Titi, whom we loved so much, our hope, our pride . . . But in such sad circumstances we must resign ourselves and think of those who are with us . . . Finally, my dear Lucien, let's work to treat our wounds. I hope that you will be strong and that you will wrap yourself up, so to speak, in your art . . . I must return to Parenteau, for cautery. I am improving, but I must persist. It is not conjunctivitis.'[38] Two years later in 1900, things had not changed: 'The grippe has left me with inflammation of the eye. Parenteau is going to cauterize me.'[39]

Shortly thereafter, Pissarro wrote: 'I am much better thanks to the cauterization which I was able to undergo. The eye has returned to its normal state and there has been no pus since yesterday. Sadly, while I am not troubled by the eye, I have had a severe pain in the kidneys, thick, red and infrequent urine, and constipation. Opium and Nux Vomica [a homeopathic medication] have stopped the constipation and probably have acted favorably on the congestion of the eye.'[40]

In 1901, Pissarro's 71st year, cauterization was continued, as had been done to him for twenty years. He died two years later in 1903.

A new era in lacrimal surgery was being developed while Pissarro was being treated by late 19th century therapeutic means. Toti, in Italy, revived ancient methods of nasal drainage, when he published his dacryocystorhinostomy procedure the year after Pissarro died (1904). Toti brought the open lacrimal sac into contact with the nasal mucosa through a bony opening. Pissarro's case history typifies Duke-Elder's comments on inflammation of the tear sac:

The history of the treatment of dacryocystitis is interesting not only because of its antiquity and the many expedients which have at various times been tried since the era of the Code of Hammurabi (c. 1800 BC) but also because it exemplifies vividly the tendency for advances in knowledge to move in circles rather than in straight lines: There are few things under the sun which are really new. The story certainly serves to show how resourceful is the ingenuity of man and how great the toleration of a sick body (Duke-Elder, 1924).

Notes

1. Bull Mem Soc Fr Ophtal, 1884–1926.
2. Rev Homoéop Fr, 1900–1935.
3. Parenteau D. Leçons de Clinique Ophtalmologique. Paris: Doin, 1881.
4. Parenteau D. Education de l'Oeil et son Hygiène. Paris: Pharmacie Centrale Homéopathique, 1889.
5. Parenteau D. Thérapeutique Homéopathique en Ophtalmologie. Paris: Doin, 1934.
6. Bailly-Herzberg J. Correspondance de Camille Pissarro, 5 vols. Paris: Valhermeil, 1988–1992. Vol. 2: pp. 270–271.
7. Ibid., Vol. 2: pp. 285–286.
8. Ibid., Vol. 3: p. 9
9. Ibid., Vol. 3: p. 13.
10. Ibid., Vol. 3: p. 18.
11. Ibid., Vol. 3: p. 51.
12. Ibid., Vol. 3: p. 70.
13. Ibid., Vol. 3: p. 73.
14. Ibid., Vol. 3: p. 73.
15. Terson A. Sur la destruction du sac au thermo-cautère et son extirpation totale dans les fistules et tumeurs lacrimales rebelles. Arch d'Ophtal. 1891; 11: 224–242.
16. Terson A. Rapport sur le traitement des affections des voies lacrimales. Bull Mem Soc Fr Ophtal, 1891; 9: 336.
17. Toti A. Nuovo metodo conservatore di cura radicale delle suppurazioni croniche del saco lacrimale (dacriocistorinostomia) La Clinica Moderna 1904; 10: 385–387.
18. Duke-Elder S, ed. System of Ophthalmology, Vol. 13: The Ocular Adnexa. St. Louis: Mosby, 1974; 714–717.
19. Correspondence, Vol. 3: pp. 74–75.
20. Ibid., Vol. 3: p. 106.
21. Ibid., Vol. 3: pp. 114–115.
22. Ibid., Vol. 3: p. 127.
23. Ibid., Vol. 3: p. 265.
24. Ibid., Vol. 3: p. 321.
25. Parenteau D. Du Massage oculaire. Bull Mem Soc Fr Ophtal 1895; 13: 456–463; Parenteau D. Kystes et gommes des paulières. Bull Mem Soc Fr Ophtal 1896; 14: 227–230.
26. Correspondence, Vol. 3: p. 321.
27. Ibid., Vol. 3: pp. 322–323.
28. Ibid., Vol. 3: pp. 324–325.
29. Ibid., Vol. 3: p. 326.
30. Ibid., Vol. 3. p. 328.
31. Ibid., Vol. 3: p. 330.
32. Ibid., Vol. 3: p. 331.
33. Ibid., Vol. 3: p. 349.
34. Ibid., Vol. 3: p. 390.
35. Ibid., Vol. 4: p. 227.

36. Ibid., Vol. 4: p. 229.
37. Ibid., Vol. 4: p. 409.
38. Ibid., Vol. 4: p. 418.
39. IBid., Vol. 5: p. 65.
40. Ibid., Vol. 5: p. 118.

Address for correspondence: James G. Ravin, MD, MS, Surgical Director, The Eye Center of Toledo, 3000 Regency Court Suite 100, Toledo, OH 43623, USA

Documenta Ophthalmologica **86**: 203–208, 1994.

Didymus the Blind: An unknown precursor of Louis Braille and Helen Keller

JOHN LASCARATOS & SPYROS MARKETOS
Department of History of Medicine, Athens University Medical School, Athens, Greece

Key words: History of Ophthalmology, Antiquity, Blindness, Louis Braille, Didymus, Helen Keller

Abstract. The present study presents the case of Didymus the Blind, worthy author, philosopher and theologian of the 4th century AD. Blinded by ophthalmia at the age of four years, Didymus succeeded in achieving great learning in the philosophical and natural sciences. He began his education by using a system which was remarkably like Braille, that is reading letters engraved into the surface of wood by touch and subsequently furthering his knowledge by listening. This learning process of Didymus the Blind appears as the precursor of Louis Braille who invented the educational system of reading embossed dots by touch. Like Didymus, Braille lost his vision in infancy (at three years of age). Another parallel of Didymus' career and written works is found in the example and achievements of Helen Keller.

Didymus the Blind, an eminent theologian of the 4th century and a student of Origen was born in Alexandria in 309 AD. He was of Greek descent. At the age of four, as the monk Palladius (ca. 368–430) writes, he was afflicted by ophthalmia and lost his sight. Thanks however to his superhuman diligence, he succeeded in achieving the highest scientific education and in so doing became the most prolific and famous scholar of the age. He was appointed to the position of Director of the Theological School of Alexandria where he taught for over fifty years, until his death in 395 or 398 [1–4].

Didymus had a profound command of the philosophic, scientific and theological theories of his time. The main sources of his material were Platonic, Aristotelian, Stoic and Neoplatonic.

He chiefly concerned himself with philosophy, in addition to poetry, rhetoric, astronomy, grammar, geometry, music and mathematics [3, 5, 7]. It is also known that he concentrated his attention on medical topics and was influenced by Hippocratic theories, although there are indications that his oeuvre is influenced by Galen's writings too [6, 8].

Further, it is interesting to note that Didymus' lessons were followed not only by the students of the Theological School of Alexandria, but that other listeners also converged en masse from all corners of the city and from other countries of the East, especially to hear and follow Didymus' famous lectures [6, 9].

Numbering amongst his pupils were the most renowned scholars of his

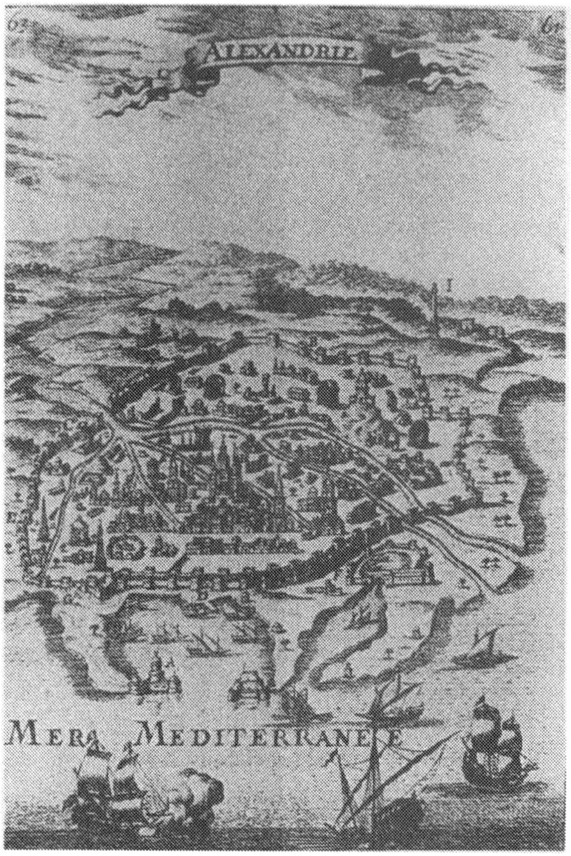

Fig. 1. An old engraving of the town of Alexandria.

age, Greeks and Latins, as for example St. Jerome (340–420), the ecclesiastic author Tyrranius Rufinus (ca. 340–410), Palladius and others.

At a young age Didymus became a monk and continued to live beyond the environs of Alexandria as a recluse. He was a fervent exponent of orthodox dogma and a supporter of St. Anthony, Athanassius the Great and other orthodox bishops in the battle against the Arian heresy.

Didymus was a most prolific author and his output, in spite of his blindness handicap can be considered extraordinary and unbelievable. He must not be confused with Didymus of Alexandria, Secretary of the Alexandrian School and critic (63 BC–10 AD) who was another extremely prolific author. Many of Didymus' works had been lost but were discovered during the Second World War at Toura, Egypt and were published under the title *Footnotes of Toura* [8, 10]. Actually his works were far greater in number and a large part of them had been lost. His writings can be generally divided into the dogmatic and the interpretive, the latter representing footnotes, as they applied to the Old and New Testaments. From the philosophical viewpoint, Didymus was an Origenist, and in essence he adopted certain unorthodox views of Origen. As is commonly understood, Origenism represents the absorption of Platonism and Neo-Platonism by the Church and Theology.

Origenism, as well as followers of its heretical views, i.e. Evagrius and Didymus, was condemned as anathema by the 5th Ecumenical Synod of Constantinople (553 AD), without however the church forbidding the reading of Didymus' works which contain orthodox views in many areas [10]. This ban was lifted after subsequent Synods [5].

Moreover, he took an active part in the counter-charges on the Holy Trinity issue, as a truly strong adversary of Arianism, and in company with Basil the Great and Saints Athanassius and Gregory, drafted the dogma of the Synod of Nicea, i.e., the consubstantiality of the Holy Spirit in relation to the other two figures of the Holy Trinity [4, 5, 10].

Didymus' enormous literary and didactic output of works must be especially highlighted as he had lost his sight at the age of four years. We do not know the exact cause, as his blindness is termed generally 'ophthalmia'. Despite the loss of his sight he succeeded in obtaining an important education in all aspects of the philosophical and natural sciences and produced an enormous literary yield. His student Rufinus writes that 'When he was small and had not yet learned the letters of the alphabet, he lost his vision, but was impassioned by the strong desire to attain true enlightenment, that being Knowledge.

Truly, through study, perspiration and nocturnal work, he profited only from hearing, where others were able to benefit by additional sight. He produced his notable works and thus in a short space of time he achieved so much education and gained so much learning of divine and earthly things that he was appointed as a professor of the Ecclesiastical School' [3].

Palladius, who also served as his student for fifteen years, notes that: 'Didymus had the misfortune, as he himself recounted (to Palladius), to lose his sight at the age of four years before he had learned to read or begun to study with tutors' [11].

The Byzantine historian Socrates the Scholastic (4th–5th century) also writes that: 'Didymus was a most admirable man and highly cultivated and was among the best, if not the best in every form of teaching. Young as he was, he fell victim to the disease of ophthalmia and he lost his vision, but God gave him the spiritual sight in place of his natural eyes and the things he was denied by lack of vision, he learned through hearing. He was extremely brilliant and pure-hearted and in this way excelled against those who were clever and had sharp natural vision' [7].

According to the same ecclesiastical author, it is also said that when Anthony the Great came to Alexandria during the time of the Emperor Valens in order to fight against the Arian heresy, he met Didymus. When the former discerned the wisdom of the man he said to him, 'Don't be sad

Didymus for the physical loss of your vision, for only your physical eyes are absent, as even flies and mosquitoes lay claim to physical sight. However, rejoice, for you have the eyes of the angels through which you can see the God' [3, 7].

The authors Nicephorus Callistus and Sozomenos provide an even more important piece of information. Hermias Sozomenos (5th century) in agreement with previous authors regarding the wisdom and breadth of Didymus' knowledge, writes that he became blind at a very early age. When he reached adolescence, he studied at schools, so that he could learn 'with the help of his hearing, but it is also said that he learned the first letters of the alphabet through his sense of touch upon their shapes which were engraved in depth on planks of wood and that the next step, the syllables and names etc., were learned by hearing and memory. This miracle was no coincidence, nor that masses of people came to Alexandria merely to see him or to hear him, because he had reached such heights in spite of the handicap of blindness' [9].

The Byzantine author Nicephorus Callistus (14th century), characterizes him as wise and verifies the information about learning his letters by feeling their shapes engraved in wood through his sense of touch. He certifies that he was an 'extraordinary sight' for the masses which came to Alexandria to hear him speak or merely to see him [6].

This last information of Sozomenos and Nicephorus Callistus proves that Didymus learned his first letters with a method which is extremely comparable to today's system of educating the blind, i.e., by utilizing a code of embossed dots, which Louis Braille (1809–1852), the famous French educator instituted [12, 13].

Braille was uniquely likened to Didymus in that he too lost his sight at the age of barely three years (through an accident). We do not know and we cannot support the contention that Braille was inspired by the system used by Didymus the Blind. Nor do we have any historical text bearing witness that Didymus the Blind's method was copied by others or used to train the blind at the various Blind Institutions of Byzantium, although this method is referred to by two well-known ecclesiastical Byzantine authors of the 5th and 14th centuries. It is certain, from this hitherto unknown information, that Didymus the Blind learned his first letters by feeling their shapes engraved on a piece of wood, i.e., through his sense of touch and subsequently supplemented his education through the help of his sense of hearing.

Clearly it follows therefore, that Didymus the Blind was a precursor of Louis Braille and Braille's method now forms the basis of educating the blind of the whole world. Concurrently Didymus also stands as the precursor of the famous American author of the turn of the 20th century Helen Keller [12, 13]. She also served as a model of a blind woman who succeeded, through persistence and patience, in helping herself in her own life, in spite of her lost vision and hearing at the age of approximately two

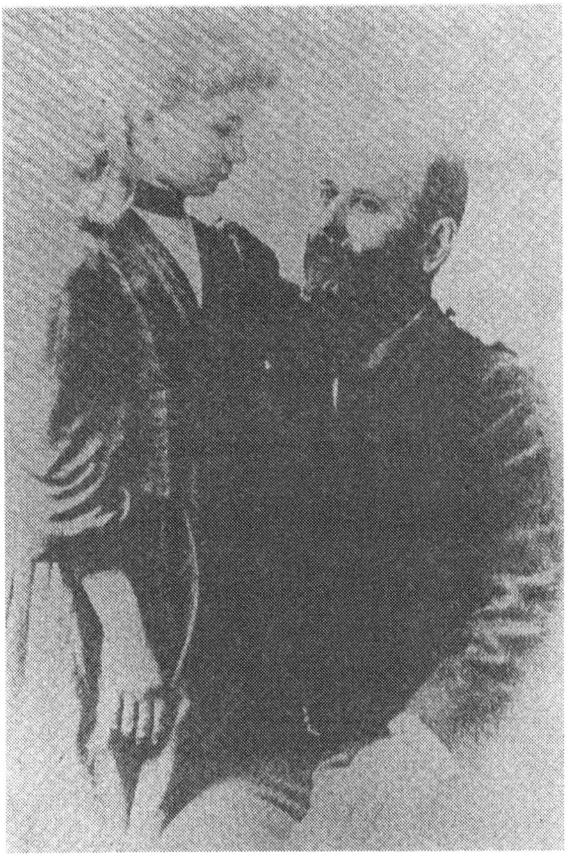

Fig. 2. Helen Keller with Michel Anagnos, Director of the School for the Blind at Boston.

years by contracting scarlet fever. With her exceptional energy and overwhelming industry she gained the broadest encyclopedic education and dedicated herself, like Didymus, to all forms of study such as philosophy, mathematics, philology, and foreign languages (including Greek and Latin) and ultimately elevated herself to such important positions as the inspector of institutions for the deaf and the dumb.

References

1. Dietsche, B. (1941–1942). L'héritage littéraire de Didyme l' Aveugle, Les Sciences Philosophiques et Théologiques, 1–2: 380–414.
2. Doutreleau, L. (1957). Le *de Trinitate* est-il l'oeuvre de Didyme l'Aveugle?, Recherches de Science Religieuse, 45: 514–557.
3. Rufini Tyrannii Aquileiensis Presbyteri, Opera Omnia etc. In: J.P. Migne (ed.) Patrologia

Latina, Vol. 21, Lib. II, Cap. VII, Vol. 516A–517A; De Didymo Alexandrino vivente. Turnhout (Belgium): Brepols.
4. S. Hieronymi, De Viris Illustribus. In: J.P. Migne (ed.) Patrologia Latina, Vol. 23, Cap. 109, Vol. 743. Turnhout (Belgium): Brepols.
5. Florafsky, G. (1964). Didymus from Alexandria, called The Blind, Religious and Moral Encyclopaedia, Vol. 4, pp. 1205–1207. Athens: A. Martinos (in Greek).
6. Nicephori Callisti, Ecclesiasticae Historiae. In: J.P. Migne (ed.), Patrologid Graeca, Vol. 146, Lib. XVII, 288 BCD. Turnhout (Belgium): Brepols.
7. Socratis, Historia Ecclesiastica. In: J.P. Migne (ed.): Patrologia Graeca. Vol. 67, Lib. IV, Cap. XXV, Col. 525 B–528 B, De Didymo Caeco. Turnhout (Belgium): Brepols.
8. Matsagas, A.K. & Marketos, S.G. (1989). Embryological concepts in Didymus teaching, Materia Medica Greca, 17 (5): 431–435 (in Greek).
9. Sozomeni Hermiae, Historia Ecclesiastica. In: J.P. Migne (ed.): Patrologia Graeca, Vol. 67, Lib. III, Cap. XV, De Didymo Caeco, et de Aetio Haeretico, Col. 1033–1034. Turnhout (Belgium): Brepols.
10. Kalamaras, M. (1973). Didymus the Blind: A treatise about the Holy Spirit. Salonica: Rigopoulos (in Greek).
11. Palladii, Helenopolitani Episcopi, Historia Lausiaca. In: J.P. Migne (ed.), Patrologia Graeca, Vol. 34. (1860), Cap. IV, 1012 D. Turnhout (Belgium): Bripols.
12. Castiglioni, A. (1947). A History of Medicine, Transl. E.B. Krumbhaar, 2nd ed. New York: A. Knopf.
13. Zahl, P.A. (1950). Blindness: Modern Approaches to the Unseen Environment. Princeton, NJ: Princeton University Press.

Address for correspondence: Prof. John Lascaratos, 9 Orinis Taxjarchias Street, Zogra fou, Athens 15772, Greece
Phone: 779 6745

Documenta Ophthalmologica **86**: 209–223, 1994.

Further ophthalmological information on Byzantine chroniclers and historians

J. FRONIMOPOULOS & J. LASCARATOS
Athens, Greece

Key words: History of Ophthalmology, Byzantium

Abstract. The historical importance of information on ophthalmological topics by Byzantine chroniclers and historians prompted us to enlarge our researches on this subject. Thus we present 17 various subjects in continuation of our previous article published in Documenta Ophthalmologica, 'History of Ophthalmology' (Vol. 5, 121–132, 1992).

Introduction

For hundreds of years Byzantium has inspired historians and in recent years Byzantine studies are to be found in the historical faculties of most universities of the world. Byzantium rose when the Roman Empire grew to include both the Greek and Christian traditions. It was an empire of Hellenism in its triumphant spread of the Greek spirit and not merely Greek blood. Thus Byzantium with its capital Konstantinou Polis (Constantinople) could resist the eastern dynasties with its ancient classical Greek tradition fortifying the spirit as a bastion of the West. Thus begins the seed of the first 'European' civilization characterized by Roman administration blended with Greek spiritual wealth.

In 1992 we published a paper concerning our findings on ophthalmological topics by Byzantine writers, mainly historians and chroniclers. The historical importance of this information prompted us to enlarge upon our researches on this subject. As most of these writers, who stem from Christian Church circles and monasteries, sought to arouse the interest of the public in religious beliefs, our findings which range from events of daily life, to narratives, describing prejudices and religious beliefs, have been grouped according to subject matter.

1. Miraculous treatments

Georgius Codinus (Pseudocodinus) (14th century AD) referring to a woman suffering from bleeding and cured by Jesus Christ miraculously, writes that she gratefully erected a statue of Christ with herself bending at the base of the statue, stretching out her hand and touching the statue.

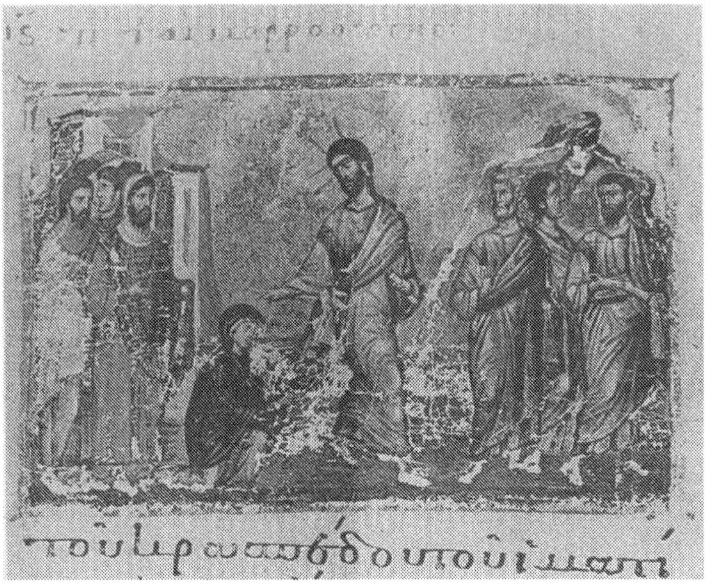

Fig. 1. The woman who was miraculously cured by Christ (Code 5, Iviron Monastery, Athos Mountain, Greece).

According to the writer, this statue was preserved till the time of Julian (361–366 AD) in the district of Panados (Fig. 1). There was a rumor, that a **herb** grew near the statue, which '**was proper** for curing every illness and especially **those people born blind**' (G. Codinus p. 177). The same miracle is mentioned by the chronicler **Malalas** (6th cent. AD–pp. 237–238). The historian **Procopius** (6th century AD), referring to the very painful gout of Augarus, governor of Edessa, during Christ's years on earth, writes that because his doctors could not help him therapeutically, he appealed to Christ Himself, who at that time was preaching to Palestine's people, and cured him miraculously. The miracles of Christ prove that he was truly the son of God for they refer to diseases incurable by the doctors of the time, as for example, the raising of the dead, cleansing those suffering from skin diseases, curing paralytics and restoring sight to those born blind (Fig. 2).

According to **Procopius**, Augurus wrote a letter asking to be cured by Him, and Christ answered in writing promising recovery; shortly thereafter he was healed (Procopius, V.I., pp. 207, 208).

2. Ophthalmic topics in the old testament

Chroniclers of world history from the dawn of time, often refer to Old Testament topics. **Ioannis Zonaras** (11th – 12th century AD) describes

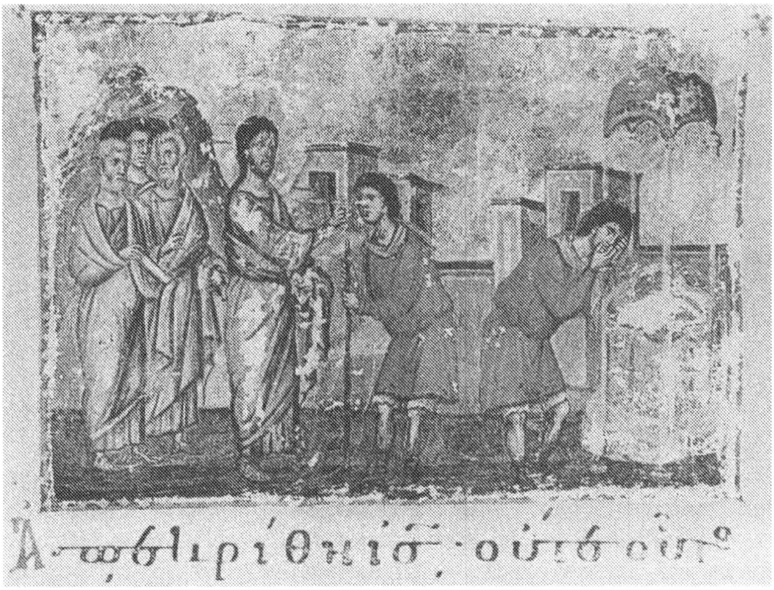

Fig. 2. Christ curing the born blind (Code 5, Iviron Monastry, Athos Mountain, Greece).

Isaac's **blindness**, probably due to eye-related retinal degenerations or senile cataract (I. Zonaras. V.I., p. 37).

The same author mentions that the Canaanite inhabitants of Jebu on the approach of King David, set up the blind, the lame and other invalids, on the battlements of the fortification's walls, to jeer at the King, thus preventing King David from entering the town. This made the King angry, and he consequently attacked and captured the town. (I. Zonaras, V.I. p. 125).

The chronicler **Georgius Cedrenus** (11th century AD) relating the Jews' history, writes that Elijah was taken up unto heaven by a whirlwind in a chariot of fire and the Lord punished the Jews by closing their eyes and making them blind; subsequently He abducted them to Samaria, where, opening their eyes, they recognized the land (G. Cedrenus I., p. 181).

The same writer mentions the punishment of Babylon's King Nebuchadnezzar, who **blinded** King Zedakiah after the capture of Jerusalem and took him to Babylon in chains. Nebuchadnezzar was punished by the Lord, who transformed his head and the front part of his body into a bull and the rest of it, into the legs of a lion. His hair grew and his nails became like those of a bird of prey and he could no longer speak. In despair he began shedding tears and his **eyes** became **'red as meat'** from weeping.

The author is probably referring to stark hyperaemia of the conjunctiva caused by crying (G. Cedrenus, I, pp. 201–204).

3. Teratogenesis

The chronicler **Michael Glycas** (12th cent. AD) describes the occurrence of teratogenesis with facts such as children born with two or three heads. Such a case occurred during the reign of Mauricius (582–602 AD). The same author remarks that some animals, eg. snakes or chickens are born with two heads or four wings and others with four paws; not however due to the influence of the stars.

Regarding these events, St. John Chrysostom, Basil the Great, Athanassius the Great, and the other Church Fathers are in accordance with the chronicler and explain **blindness at birth** or lameness at birth as afflictions due to natural causes and refute those who believe in the influence of the stars as a cause. They prefer to leave them in their ignorance, because the reason for teratogenesis is well known and often could be seen at the birth of children with anomalies, who emerged stricken from the womb.

According to Glycas, for Siamese twins to occur, the two embryos in the womb could not separate and remained stuck together. He ignores the theory of influence of the stars, originating in old Assyro-Babylonian medicine and reaching us through Renaissance literature (M. Glycas pp. 54–55).

The same chronicler describes the birth of monsters in Constantinople, during the reign of Mauricius in detail. At that time a child was born without eyes and arms and with a fish-tail. In the same town a dog was born with a lion's head and six paws; while two children were born in Thrace, one with four feet and the other with two heads. During the same period, two human-shaped animals, were born in the Nile region, hermaphrodites in fact, but termed sirens by Glycas. This phenomenon was thought to portend evil for the towns where they were born (M. Glycas, p. 507).

The above information is a sequel to those of the chroniclers mentioned in our preceding paper.

4. Amblyopia from tortures

The historian **Procopius** (6th cent. AD) writes that (Fig. 3) Justinian's (527–565 AD) wife Theodora (Fig. 4) believed that certain officers were slandering her and he summoned one of them, Bousi by name, to the palace. Although he was descended nobly from Hypatus, she had him imprisoned in a dungeon beneath the palace. There he remained, in darkness, isolated completely from human intercourse and forbidden conversation even with the guards or those who brought him food. The result was his losing the sense of time completely and when he was finally released after two years and four months, he was suffering from **amblyopia** and phylasthenia (Procopius, V III, Histor, Arcana, pp. 30, 31).

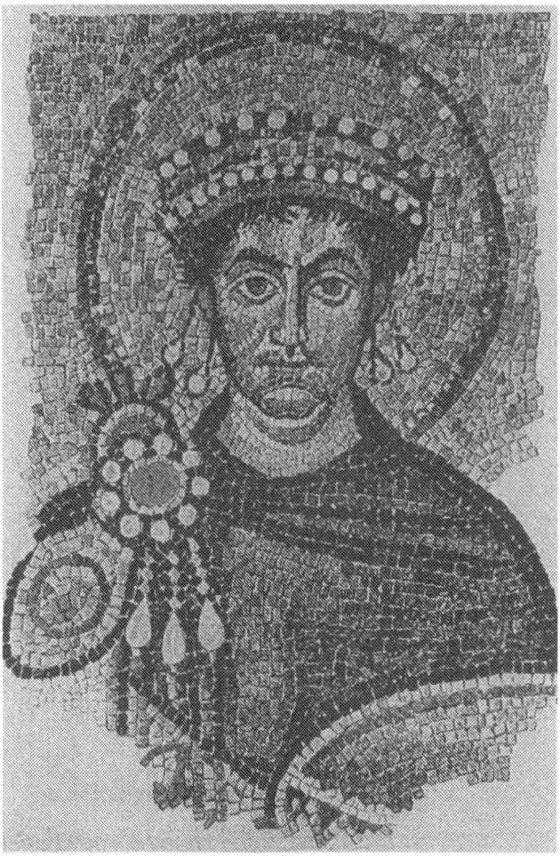

Fig. 3. The emperor Justinian I, 527–565 AD (Mosaic 6th century in the church of St. Vitalius, Ravenna, Italy).

5. Ophthalmic symptoms in general diseases

The chronicler **Georgius Cedrenus** (11th century AD) referring to Ioannis Tsimiskis' (969–976 AD) (Fig. 5) disease, considers it due to poisoning, which at its late stage presented an anthrax pimple on the shoulders and **blood flow from his eyes** (G. Cedrenus, V II p. 415). The blood flow of the eyes, if it was due to Tsimiskis being poisoned, probably resulted from the rupture of the conjunctival vessels (hyposphagma) due to high blood pressure and due to the poison aconition or to another alcoloid from herbs favoured at this time by poisoners.

The historian **Michael Psellos** (11th century AD) referring to Michael IV's (1034–1041 AD) epileptic crises, describes the precursory symptoms as: **divergence of the eyes** and the movements of the head. When this occurred

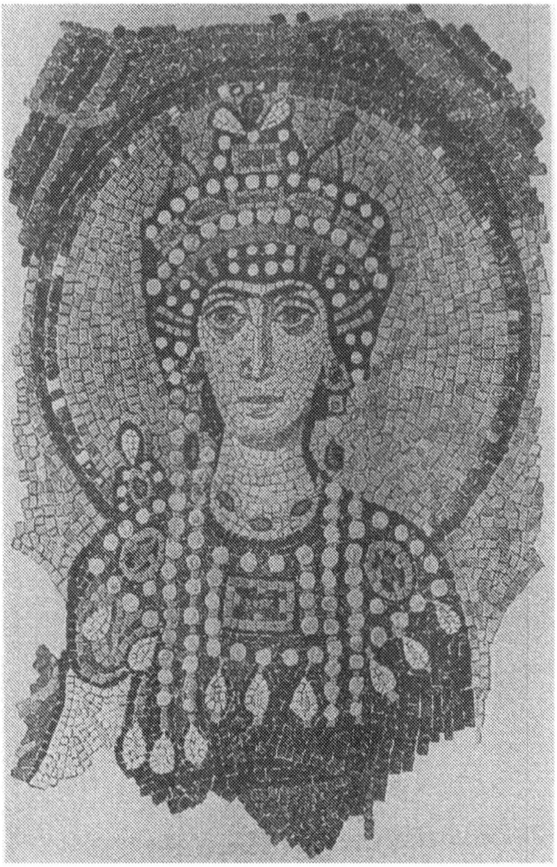

Fig. 4. Justinian's wife Theodora, 521–548 AD (Mosaic 6th century in the church of St. Vitalis, Ravenna, Italy).

his servants hurried to draw the curtain so that his subjects could not see the King during the crisis (M. Psellos, V.I., p. 63).

The historian **Michael Attaliata** (11th cent. AD) referring to Isaac I Comnenos (1057–1059 AD) writes that when the King was occupied with hunting or military exercises, **he saw a flash of light**, which struck him and he died on arrival to the palace (M. Attaliata, p. 69). **Ioannis Zonaras** (11th century AD) states two reasons for the emperor's death; the one being pleurisy and the other the epileptic crisis during a ride, when the king **saw a flash of light**, fell from his horse and began to foam at the mouth (J. Zonaras, V. III, pp. 672, 673).

Michael Glycas also refers to the **flash of light** which caused the king's fall from his horse (M. Glycas, pp. 603–604) and Ioannis Scylitzas, pp. 647–648, Efrem V. I, pp. 114, verses 3284–3293 and Ioel p. 64).

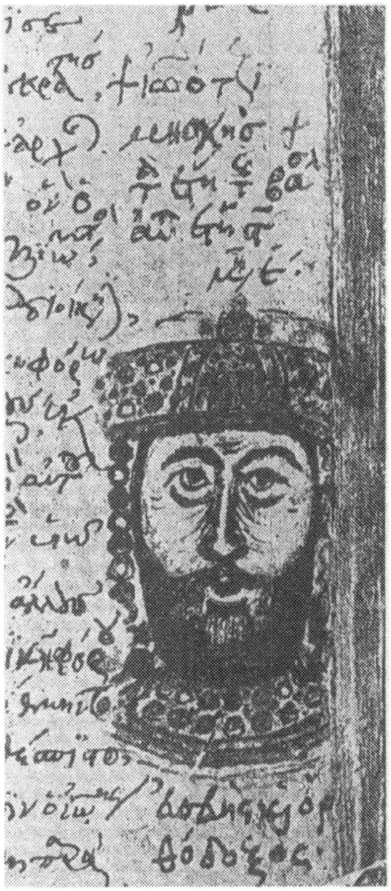

Fig. 5. The emperor Joannis Tsimiskis, 969–976 AD (Miniature 14th–15th century AD, Code α, S.5, Bibliotheca Estensa, Modena, Italy).

It is clear from these chronicles that a **flash of light** was the prodromal symptom of the epileptic crisis.

The historian **Nicephorus Callistus**, (14th cent.) describes the great epidemic plague which broke out in Justinian's reign, remarking that in many cases the disease began from the head displaying the symptoms **hyperaemic eyes** and oedema of the face (N. Callisti, V. 147, Chap. 18, coloms 265–266).

The historian **Evagrius** (6th century AD) also describes this epidemic and writes it commonly starts from the head, with bleeding eyes (Evagrius, p. 78)

A. Gabrielides recognizes this epidemic's hyperaemic eyes as hemorragic **conjunctivitis** (A. Gabrielides 1925). **Nicephorus Gregoras** (14th cent. AD) describes his own disease, with its symptoms; pain in the head, mainly localized in the eyes, from which he was suffering badly (N. Gregoras, V. III, p. 132).

6. Vitamin A deficiency

Nicephorus Callistus referring to an epidemic of famine and plague, writes that after the famine, an uncommon disease appeared named anthrax, inciting a badly smelling ulcer, located on the **inner canthus of the eyes** and resulting in blindness in both men and women. The long term result of the famine was followed by characteristic symptoms of Vitamin A deficiency (Patrologia Greca, V. 145, colomes 1268–1269).

7. Migraine

Theophanes the historian (8th–9th cent. AD) mentions a characteristic instance in the year 6256 (anus moundi, 747 AD) when the Turks returned to the Caspiae Pylae and Iberia and fought the Arabs. According to Theophanes, an Arab leader named Ise, pretender of the throne, had an attack of **migraine headache with scotoma.** Abdullah (Abdullah – Abou Ja'far Abd Allah ben Mohammed al Mancour billah) – the second calif of Damascus, family of Abbasid, seeing the illness, thought to overcome him with guile. Thus he convinced him that he would be cured by inhaling a sneezing remedy prepared by a doctor names Moses, (Ibn Mousa) deacon of the Church of Antioch, whom he had previously bribed to prepare a poison with a heavy narcotic quality. He inhaled this drug and was unconscious for three days. During these three days, Abdullah's son, Monan (or Ai-Mahdi) reigned. From this anecdote of Theophanes' we learn that doctors knew that scotoma followed migraine and we have the first written reference to a drug being inhaled (Theophanes, pp. 672–673 AD).

8. Metamorphopsy

Nicephorus Gregoras (14th cent.) writes that when you look at the blinding light of the sun at noon and then you turn away and look down at the earth again, the result is a series of images displaying different colours, which though untrue, seem to be real to the eyes (N. Gregoras, V. III, p. 320 and Gabrielides 1934).

9. Conjunctivitis from dust

The chronicler **Zosimos** (5th century AD) writes in reference to a battle of the Roman army against Skythae, that a storm arose and the horses drawing against the Skythae, raised a cloud of dust, which **damaged the soldier's eyes** (Zosimos, pp. 153). The Byzantine doctors, mainly Alexander Trallianus, were aware of the effect of dust on the eyes, and they considered it a cause of **chronic conjunctivitis** (Neuburger 1910).

10. Cataract

Ioannis Zonaras describing the **blindness** of the Bishop of Carthage, Mari, writes that, when Mari faced the emperor Julian the Apostate he called him 'evil demon' and 'denier of Christ'. The emperor pretending to be hard-hearted said: 'Go out of here, miserable man and weep for your own **blindness**'. According to Zonaras, the Bishop who was blinded from **hypochysis** answered: 'I thank Christ the Saviour who has graciously prevented me from seeing your shameless and disrespectful face.' (I. Zonaras. V. III. pp. 62–63).

According to **Nicephorus Gregoras** it is possible that the grandfather of King Andronicus the Younger (Palaeologus, 1328–1341 AD) was suffering from the same disease as Mari or from another **blinding eye disease**, and that he lost first the vision of one eye and later of the second. He remained in darkness and had to be guided to perform his duties (N. Gregoras, V.I., pp 431–446). **Georgius Pachymeres** (13th–14th cent. AD) refers to **a very bad eye disease** suffered by the Patriarch during the reign of Andronicus II Palaeologus (1282–1328 AD) (Fig. 6). The Patriarch was in Silyvria suffering from **ophthalmia**, and following the doctor's advice, was obliged to leave the town. He was transferred to the Monastery of Cosmidium for treatment. (G. Pachymeres, V. II, p. 283).

11. Similarities

The chronicler **Nicephorus Gregoras** states that certain inconsistent views must be considered ridiculous, for example the promises given by **a blind man**, to cure **the blindness** of another blind person (N. Gregoras V. II, p. 792).

12. The blindness of the General Vardas Skleros

The chronicler **Georgius Cedrenus** writes that General Vardas Skleros, (Fig. 7) who revolted against the emperor Basil II (976–1025 AD) (Fig. 8), finally declared allegiance to the King. He was honoured with the title 'Kouropalatis'. On his way to Constantinople to meet the King, **he was stricken** by blindness and was taken to the King in this condition. As the King faced him, he said with irony to those present: 'Look at the man of whom I was afraid. Now he comes to me **blind** guided by hand' (G.

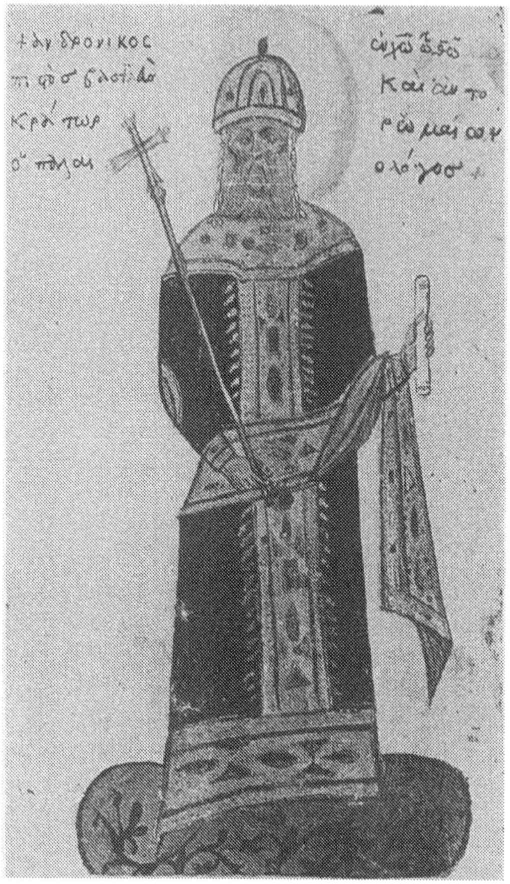

Fig. 6. The emperor Andronicus II, Paleologus, 1282–1328 (Chronicle Pachimeris, Bavarian National Library, Munich, Germany).

Cedrenus, V. II, pp. 446–447). The successor of **Joannis Skytitzae** (Continuatus, p. 339) also refers to this acute **blindness** of Vardas (989 AD) probably due to an acute **eye disease** like neuritis, thrombosis of the central artery etc).

13. Eye purchase

The anonymous writer of the 'Epirotica' cites a curious **eye purchase**, recalling the practice of bailing out slaves. In 1380 the Turks captured the Abbot of Metzovo Isaias and put him in jail. They decided to **blind** him but some clever and loyal Christians, knowing the avarice of the Turks

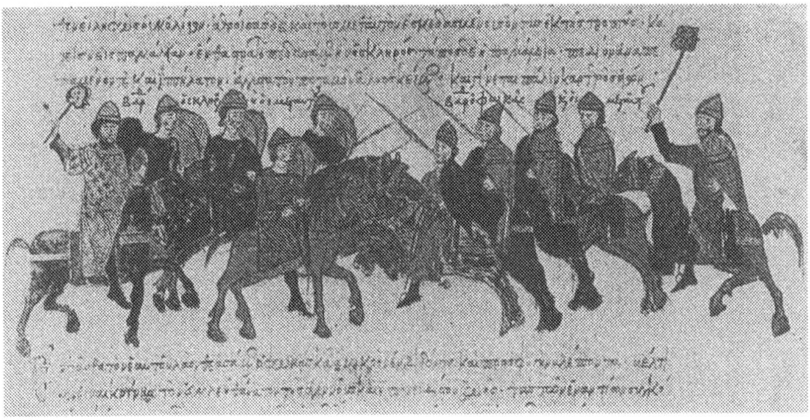

Fig. 7. General Vardas Skleros (left) in a battle against Vardas Phokas (right), 976–985 (Chronicle J. Skilitsis, National Library, Madrid, Spain).

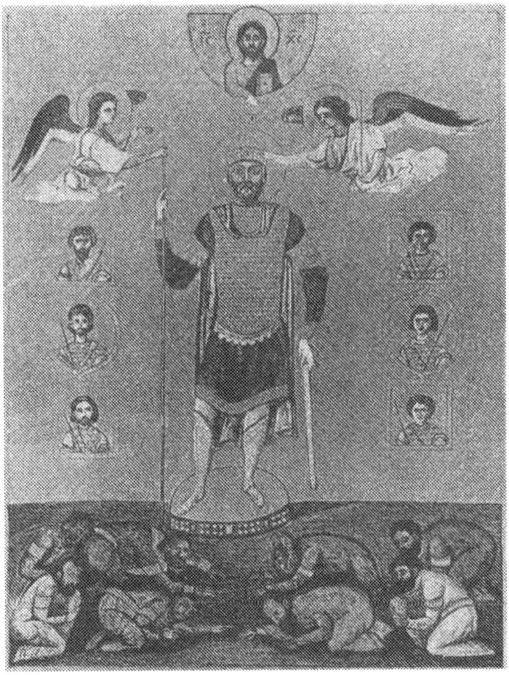

Fig. 8. The emperor Basil II, Boulgaroktonos, 976–1025 AD (Miniature 11th century, Code XIII, Bibliotheca Marciana, Venice, Italy).

'purchased his eyes' for 200 aspra. But even so, the Turks enucleated the eyes of the Abbot and burned him (Epirotica, pp. 227–228).

14. Prejudices relevant to contagious eye diseases

The chronicler **Melitinos** (10th century AD) imparts important information about the plague which appeared in the Roman empire during the reign of Gallus and Valusianus. The plague which lasted 11 years started from both East and West and no towns escaped from the fear of contamination. According to this author, the disease was transferred via clothes and via **the Eye** (Melitinos, p. 57). This was a common prejudice which, like others, prevailed during these years.

According to the chronicler **Glycas**, contamination from eye diseases is transferred through the air, when someone looks at a suffering person (Gabrielides 1956). This view, i.e. that infections are transferred through the air, is similar to the theories of Aristotle, Alexander Aphrodisieus and Plutarch.

Glycas referring to swallows, writes that mothers cure their nestlings when suffering from **ophthalmia**, by smearing their eyes with some substance (Glycas, p. 79 and Gabrielides 1936). He also writes about the vision of fish which is poor and the eagle, which is very sharp and endures the sun's brightness (Glycas p. 80).

15. Aetiology of eye diseases

According to **St. John Chrysostom** the **amblyopias** as well as the pain in the arms and feet and also fevers are not due to malnutrition but to greediness and to excesses (Migne, P.G., V. 59 col 1,57).

The chronicler **Nikitas Choniates** (12–13th cent.) writes that the outbreak of diseases such as fever, arthritis, **eye infections**, coincides with the summer months and recedes during the winter time (N. Choniates, V. III, pp. 114–115).

16. Dicoria (Iris heterochromia)

The Byzantine writers use the term **'dicoria'** for the **heterochromia** of the iris. The chronicler **Malalas** referring to the emperor Anastasios I (491–518 AD) (Fig. 9) writes that he had normal eyes, but **the irises were of different colours**, the right eye being light blue and the left dark (Malalas. p. 392).

Michael Glycas also refers to the **dicoria** of Emperor Anastasios A'Dirrachinos and describes his eyes, the right iris being blue and the left iris dark. The description is similar to Malalas' description (M. Glycas, p. 491).

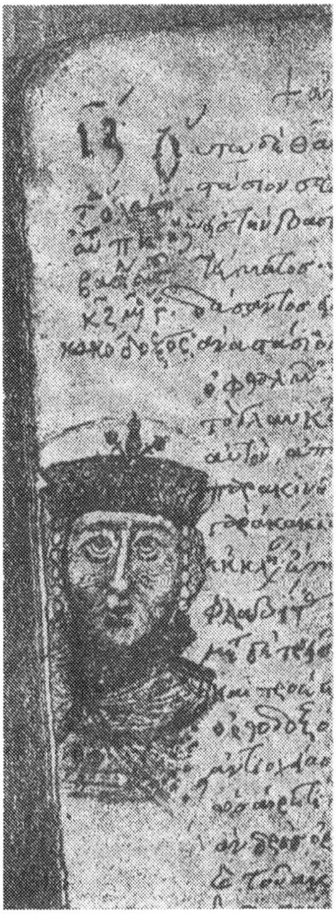

Fig. 9. The emperor Anastasios, 491–518 AD (Code α S 5.5, Bibliotheca Estensa, Modena, Italy).

The chronicler **Konstantinos Mannasses** (12 cent. AD) (Fig. 10) also referring to the **heterochromia** of the emperor Anastasios, writes about it in verses (Manasses p. 130, verses 3009-3011). The bishop **Dorotheos of Monemvasia** (15th cent.) also describes Anastasios as **'dicoros'**, because one of the irises was green and the other dark (Gabrielides 1936).

17. The blindness of the Apostle Paul

The chronicler **Michael Glycas** referring to the **blindness** of the Apostle Paul writes that during his course to Damascus a flash of light burst over his head with an indescribable light and thus 'the lanterns of his eyes were extinguished'. Paul later regained his sight by accepting baptism and regained both his physical and spiritual vision (Glycas pp. 423–424). An explanation of Paul's blindness is given by A. Gabrielides (1933).

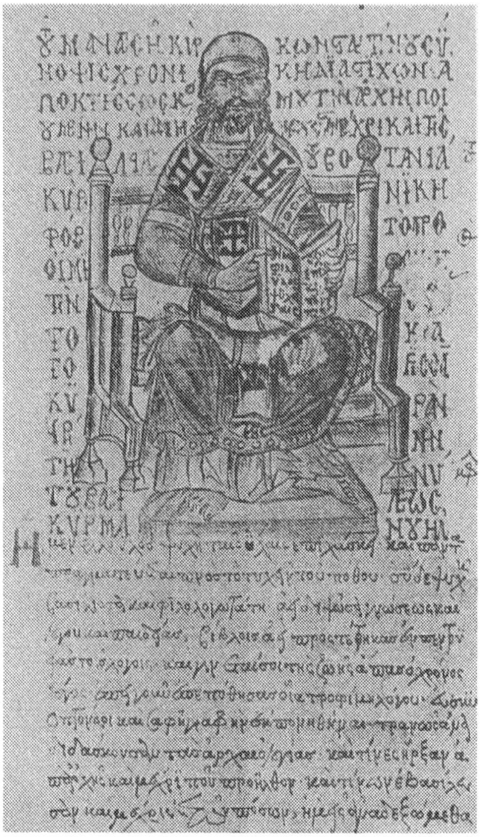

Fig. 10. The chronicler Constantinus Manasses (Miniature 14th century, National Library, Vienne, Austria).

Conclusions

The Byzantine historians and chroniclers by providing us with interesting ophthalmological information, enrich our medical knowledge of this period.

The history of medicine in the 19th and 20th century became a critical science, using the inheritance of historical sources and the experience of the past, not for a barren encyclopedic education, but as a means through which to analyze in a critical way, the evolution and the course of medicine through the disciplines of sociology and philosophy. This proves how valuable the researches and historical studies from books and medical articles are. Byzantine medicine influenced by Hippocratic, Alexandrian and Roman teachings succeeded, after the fall of the Byzantine empire, in being transferred to Europe, thus contributing to the medical knowledge of the Renaissance period.

Bibliography

1. **Nicephori Callisti**, Ecclesiasticae Historiae, Migne Patrologia Graeca (P.G.), Vol. 145, Lib. VII, Cap. XXVIII, Colomes 1268–1269 Vol. 147, Lib. XVII, Cap, XVIII, volumes 265–266.
2. The 13 references of the authors correspond to the Volumes of the **Corpus Scriptorum Historiae Byzantinae**. Editio emendatior et Copriosior, consilio B.G. Niebuhrii C.F. (50 volumes Bonnae, E. Weberi, 1828–1897):
   1) Michael Attaliota
   2) Georgius Cedrenus, Vol I, II – Ioannes Curopalatae (Skylitzae).
   3) Georgius Codinos (Pseudocodinos)
   4) Michael Glycas
   5) Nicephorus Gregoras, Vol. I, II, III.
   6) Malalas
   7) Constantinus Manassas, Ioel, Georgius Acropolita
   8) Georgius Pachymeres, Vol. II
   9) Procopius, Vol. I, III
   10) Theophanes, Vol I
   11) Ioannis Zonaras, Vol I
   12) Zosimus
   13) Historia Politica et Patriarchica Constantinopoleos, Epirotica.
3. **Corpus Fontium Historiae Byzantinae**
   a) **Ioannis Scylitzae**, Synopsis Historiarum, Recensuit Ioannes Thurm, Walter de Gruyter et Socios, Berolini et Novi Eboraci, 1973.
   b) **Nicetae Choniatae** Orationes et Epistulae, Recensuit I. – **A. Van Dieten, Walter de Gruyter et Socios**, Berolini **et Novi** Eboraci, 1972. (Series Berolinensis, vol III, Ed H.-G. Beck – A. Hambylis – R. Keydell).
4. **S. Ioannis Chrysostomi, Archiep. Constantinop.**, Migne, P.G., vol 59, colome 157.
5. **Efraim of Aevias**. Chronography, Vol. A-B, Translation-Comments Od. Lampsidis, Edit Center of Greek writers, Athens 1984.
6. **Evagrius**, The Ecclesiastical History, Ed. J. Bidez and L. Parmentier. Amsterdam, A.M. Hakkert. 1964.
7. **Gabrielides A**. (1925) The plague by Byzantine Writers. Bull. Med. Soc. of Athens pp. 39–40.
8. **Gabrielides A**. (1933) Ophthalmics in the Acts of the Apostles. Bull. Gr. Ophth. Soc. 227–243.
9. **Gabrielides A**. (1934) Photoplexy by the Ancients. Bull. Gr. Ophth. Soc., 27–34.
10. **Gabrielides A**. (1936) Ophthalmological Knowledge by Kyros Michael Glycas. Bull. Gr. Ophth. Soc. 51–71.
11. **Theodosii Meliteni**, Chronographia, Ed. Th. Tafel, Monachii 1859, G. Franz.
12. **Neuburger M**. (1910) History of Medicine, vol. I, Transl. E. Prayfair, London, H. Frowde, Hodder and Stoughton.
13. **Psellos Michael**, Chronographie, Vol I, Texte établi et traduit par Emile Renaud, Paris, Société d'Edition 'Les Belles Lettres', 1967.
14. **Fronimopoulos J., Lascaratos J**., Some Byzantine Chroniclers and Historians on Ophthalmological Topics, Documenta Ophthalmologica 81(1), History of Ophthalmology Vol. 5, 121–132, 1992.

A THREE-LINGUAL PUBLICATION IN ENGLISH, FRENCH AND GERMAN

A. BRINI / P. DHERMY / J. SAHEL

Oncology of the Eye and Adnexa

ATLAS OF CLINICAL PATHOLOGY

The authors have put together, side by side, clinical and histopathological aspects of the various neoformations likely to be encountered in eye pathology, including those most recently discovered as well as those most frequently met with. The aim of the authors is to provide their colleagues with a reference MANUAL, conceived so as to permit rapid access to essential concepts in current eye oncology. Rapid and easy consultation of this atlas has been made possible through the use of a comprehensive set of 64 plates, with 375 full-colour figures, with concise accompanying texts in English, French and German, and a detailed index.

From the Contents:

A. Tumours of the eylids and the conjuctiva / Tumeurs palpébro-conjonctivales / Geschwülste der Augenlider und der Bindehaut
B. Orbital and orbito-palpebral tumours / Tumeurs de l'orbite et orbito-palpébrales / Orbitale und orbito-palpebrale Geschwülste
C. Tumours of the uvea / Tumeurs de l'uvée / Geschwülste der Uvea
D. Tumours of the retina and the optic disc / Tumeurs de la rétine et de la papille optique / Geschwülste der Netzhaut und der Papille

Technical appendix / Appendice technique / Technischer Anhang
Literature / Littérature / Literatur
Alphabetical index of subjects / Index des sujets / Sachwörterverzeichnis

Not only students beginning with work in ophthalmology, but also experienced ophthalmologists will find this atlas most useful. At the same time, it should be considerable assistance to pathologists and dermatologists and to practitioners frequently finding themselves faced with ophthalmological problems.

XX + 154 pages with 375 colour-photographs HB ISBN 0-7923-0409-8

A PUBLICATION OF
Kluwer Academic Publishers - Dordrecht / Boston / London

A Short History of Breast Cancer

The frequency of breast cancer seems to be on the increase since about the middle of the 19th century. This does not mean, however, that the disease was not encountered before. It was already mentioned together with cancer of the skin and the uterus in the Hippocratic writings earlier than the fourth century B.C.
Although mammary cancer has been studied for some 25 centuries, its cause is still largely unknown. Despite the huge amounts of money spent on cancer research, the intensive efforts of innumerable scientists all over the world and the advanced technology of modern medicine, there has been no substantial improvement in therapeutic results in recent decades, and there still exists no uniformity of approach regarding the best method of treatment. It was felt that a review of the main pathogenic concepts and therapeutic principles regarding breast cancer, placed in the context of the development of medicine in general over the course of Western civilization, might contribute to a better understanding of where we stand today.

From the Contents: (1) Antiquity, (2) The Middle Ages, (3) The Renaissance, (4) Patho-physiological concepts in the Age of the Enlightenment, (5) Diagnosis and therapy in the 18th century, (6) Europe during Napoleon and after, (7) Scientific developments in the second half of the 19th century, (8) Mammary carcinoma in the light of new developments, (9) Surgical treatment in the second half of the 19th century, (10) The 20th century – Epilogue – Notes – Index of names.

1983, xiv + 124 pages – with 39 photographs. ISBN 0-89828-562-8

A History of Surgery

This book consists of original research into development of surgery through the ages and provides a chronological survey of the events which have lead to the modern achievements in surgery. There is an emphasis on surgical practice within the Netherlands. Dutch surgery, however, has by no means been taken as a phenomenon: it is considered in its context within European surgery as a whole, whilst contemporary medical thinking is set against a cultural and political background.

From the Contents: (1) The roots of Western surgery, (2) The Western Middle Ages, (3) The Renaissance, (4) The Golden Age, (5) The Age of Enlightenment, (6) Practical surgery in the 17th and 18th centuries, (7) The beginning of modern surgery, (8) Antisepsis: a turning point in surgery, (9) The German period in Dutch surgery, (10) Surgery in the past 75 years – Notes – Bibliography – Index of names

1988, xxiv + 408 pages – with 127 illustrations. ISBN 0-89838-968-2

About the author. After a career as an active surgeon Daniel de Moulin switched to medical history and he was Professor of the History of Medicine at the Catholic University, Nijmegen, The Netherlands.

Both volumes contain many historical illustrations, most of them not previously published.

KLUWER ACADEMIC PUBLISHERS – DORDRECHT / BOSTON / LONDON

www.ingramcontent.com/pod-product-compliance
Ingram Content Group UK Ltd.
Pitfield, Milton Keynes, MK11 3LW, UK
UKHW020239160926
475610UK00001B/64
* 9 7 8 0 7 9 2 3 3 1 0 1 8 *